Resistance Band Workout for Seniors

Improve Energy, Mobility, and Vitality with This Easy to Read Guide

Francis Papun

© Copyright 2020 - All rights reserved.

The content contained within this book may not be reproduced, duplicated or transmitted without direct written permission from the author or the publisher.

Under no circumstances will any blame or legal responsibility be held against the publisher, or author, for any damages, reparation, or monetary loss due to the information contained within this book, either directly or indirectly.

Legal Notice:

This book is copyright protected. It is only for personal use. You cannot amend, distribute, sell, use, quote, or paraphrase any part, or the content within this book, without the consent of the author or publisher.

Disclaimer Notice:

Please note the information contained within this document is for educational and entertainment purposes only. All effort has been executed to present accurate, up to date, reliable, complete information. No warranties of any kind are declared or implied. Readers acknowledge that the author is not engaged in the rendering of legal, financial, medical, or professional advice. The content within this book has been derived from various sources. Please consult a licensed professional before attempting any techniques outlined in this book.

By reading this document, the reader agrees that under no circumstances is the author responsible for any losses, direct or indirect, that are incurred as a result of the use of the information contained within this document, including, but not limited to, errors, omissions, or inaccuracies.

SPECIAL BONUS!

Get this additional Free 30 Days to Fitness Challenge Book 100% FREE!

Hundreds of others are already enjoying insider access to all of my current and future full-length books, 100% free!

If you want insider access plus this Free 30 Days to Fitness Challenge Book, all you have to do is **scan the code below** with your smartphone camera to claim your offer!

Table of Contents

INTRODUCTION 1

    How Will This Book Benefit Me? 3
    Who Is the Author? 4
    Benefits of Regular Exercise for Seniors 6
    My Promise to You 8
    But...You Have to Act! 9

CHAPTER 1: WHAT IS RESISTANCE TRAINING? 11

    How Exactly Does the Body Build Muscle? 11
    Why Are Bands a Good Choice? 13
    Making the Right Choice 15
    The Top 10 Resistance Band Training Rules 16
    The Bottom Line 20

CHAPTER 2: HEALING FROM INJURY 23

    Common Injuries Healed With Resistance Training 23
        Shoulder Dislocation or Pain 24
        Tennis Elbow 24
        Runner's Knee 25
        Hip Bursitis 25
        Sprains and Strains 26
        Recovery After Knee-Repair Surgery 26
    Phases of Recuperation After Injury 27
        Reaction Phase 27
        Regeneration 28
        Remodeling Stage 28
    A Note of Caution 29
    Breathe, Breathe, Breathe 29
        In and Out 30
        Belly Breathing 31
    Consistency Is Key 32

- THE ROLE OF GENETICS 33
  - *Ectomorphs...33*
  - *Endomorphs..34*
  - *Ectomorphs...34*
- TYPES OF RESISTANCE BANDS 35
  - *Mini Bands..35*
  - *Tubing..36*
- THE RESISTANCE LEVEL 37
  - *How to Find the Right Level 37*
  - *Adjusting Resistance During an Exercise 38*
- DO YOU NEED MORE CONVINCING?..................................39

CHAPTER 3: WARM-UPS AND STRETCHES 41

- SUGGESTED EXERCISES 42
  - *Windmill Exercise...42*
  - *Elbow Touch...43*
  - *Tennis Elbow Warm-Up 43*
  - *Shoulder Box Exercise 44*
  - *Choker Exercise 45*
  - *Wrist Stretch..46*
  - *Knee to Chest Exercise 47*
  - *Sit & Reach Exercise 48*
  - *Rear Calf Stretch Exercise 49*
  - *Gas Pedal Exercise 49*
  - *Twister Exercise...50*
  - *Side Bend Exercise...51*
  - *Rock 'n Roll Exercise..51*
  - *Head Lift Exercise..52*
  - *Tennis Watcher Exercise 53*

CHAPTER 4: UNDERSTANDING THE BENEFITS OF STRENGTH TRAINING 55

- STRENGTH TRAINING IN A NUTSHELL 56
  - *Strength Training and Diseases 58*
  - *Increasing Anaerobic Endurance 60*
  - *The Cardiovascular and Pulmonary Systems 61*
- A SOLUTION FOR THE WHOLE BODY..................................61
- AN "ANTI-AGING FORMULA" 62

FACTORS AFFECTING SUCCESS 63
   Nutrition 63
HOW TO AVOID THE WEIGHT LOSS STALL 66
   Body Composition 67

CHAPTER 5: TYPES OF RESISTANCE BANDS AND SPECIFICATIONS 69

LOOP RESISTANCE BANDS 70
   O-Shaped Expanders 71
TUBE RESISTANCE BANDS 71
   Thermoplastic Rubber 73
   Extruded Rubber 73
   Latex 74
MINI HIP CIRCLE RESISTANCE BANDS 75
RENRANRING RESISTANCE BANDS 75
FIGURE 8 RESISTANCE BANDS 76
LETSFIT RESISTANCE POWER LOOP BANDS 76
THERAPY BANDS 77
   Theraband Resistance Therapy Bands 78
   Whatafit Resistance Therapy Bands 78
   Perfect Peach Resistance Therapy Bands 79
TRIBE RESISTANCE BANDS 79
VALEO RESISTANCE BANDS 79
EDX RESISTANCE BANDS 80
LUX FITNESS RESISTANCE BANDS 80
ZIFTEX RESISTANCE BANDS 81
PHYSIOWORKS RESISTANCE BANDS 81
8-SHAPE RESISTANCE BANDS 81
BFR BANDS 83
   Superpump BFR bands 83
RESISTANCE BAND ROLLERS 84
FOAM ROLLERS 84
PULL-UP BANDS 86
LONG BANDS 86
KINETIC LEG RESISTANCE STRAPS 87
DOOR ANCHORS 87
ANKLE STRAPS 88
HANDLES 88

CHAPTER 6: RESISTANCE BAND SERIES EXERCISES 91

THE MAIN BODY PARTS 91
- Upper Body 92
- Lower Body 99
- The Core 102
- The Back 103
- The Abdominal Area 105

GOLFING EXERCISES 108
- Targeted Warm-Ups 108
- Joint Stability..109
- The All-Important Swing 109
- Fitness 110

ADDING ACCESSORIES 111
- Balls 112
- Dumbbells..113

CHAPTER 7: SAMPLE CORE WORKOUTS 115

CORE WORKOUT 1 115
- Bicycle Crunch 116
- Mountain Climber...116
- Hip Thrust 117

CORE WORKOUT 2 117
- Low-High Chop..118
- Side Plank Row..118
- High Leg Raise...119
- High Plank Row...119

CORE WORKOUT 3 120
- Bicycle Crunch 120
- Mountain Climber...120
- Torso Rotation 121
- Side Plank Reach...122

OTHER EXERCISES TO MIX AND MATCH 122

CHAPTER 8: DESIGNING YOUR OWN PROGRAMS............... 127

TWO WORKOUTS PER WEEK PROGRAM......................................127
- Day One 127
- Day Two 130

- THREE WORKOUTS PER WEEK PROGRAM 132
  - *Day One* *132*
  - *Day Two* *134*
  - *Day Three* *135*
- FOUR WORKOUTS PER WEEK PROGRAM 136
  - *Day One* *136*
  - *Day Two* *137*
  - *Day Three* *138*
  - *Day Four* *138*
- BEGINNER FIVE OR SIX DAY WORKOUT 139
  - *Day One* *140*
  - *Day Two* *140*
  - *Day Three* *141*
  - *Day Four* *141*
  - *Day Five* *142*
  - *Day Six* *142*
- ADVANCED FIVE OR SIX DAY WORKOUT 143
  - *Day One* *143*
  - *Day Two* *144*
  - *Day Three* *145*
  - *Day Four* *145*
  - *Day Five* *146*
  - *Day Six* *147*

CONCLUSION **149**

- A FINAL PIECE OF ADVICE 150

REFERENCES **151**

IMAGES **178**

Introduction

"Aging is not lost youth, but a new stage of opportunity and strength." — Betty Friedan, Author and Activist

Sarah was telling her friends about her attempt at exercising at the age of 68. "I got permission from my doctor to join the fitness group. The first time I jumped, gyrated, huffed, and puffed for over an hour. By the time I got my leotard on, it was past the class's starting time!"

Fitness and mobility do not have to be such elusive goals for seniors. It may seem hard to believe that anyone battling decreasing suppleness and lamenting their level of fitness can maintain a routine the same as when they were younger.

Is getting up in the morning harder than it used to be? Are your joints achy and stiff, and is bending down to pick something up a major issue? Are you afraid of going downstairs because you don't feel confident in your balance? Does your list of chronic medications keep getting longer?

Do you suffer from anxiety attacks and depression because you fear losing your independence and mobility? Do you miss the overall good feeling of having exercised your body and being rid of all the creaks and pains that sometimes seem to appear overnight?

If the idea of going to a gym to get moving again is even scarier than the possible consequences of doing no exercise at all, this book is here to help. Packed full of information about training without risk of injury while maximizing strength and therapeutic benefits, and staying in your own home to boot, the book is a treasure trove of helpful exercises. You will see how easy it is to get your fitness and health back with only minimal equipment required, and objects already in your home. It is simple and economical - an elegant solution to a health problem.

The information can be taken with you wherever you travel, so you never have to miss any training session on account of being in a hotel or on vacation. Resistance bands are lightweight and compact and you will learn how to choose your purchases wisely to make a wide variety of exercises possible with only a few different bands.

Each exercise has been discussed in detail and all care was taken to describe them as plainly as possible. Most of the exercises have been adapted to standing or sitting positions. Skip those that have to be done lying down on the floor especially if your body is not comfortable in this position, or try to modify them for more comfortable surfaces to lie on. While your workout should challenge you, it should never be painful; listen to your body to achieve the best results. You should not exercise to the point of collapsing after the last repetition.

Be sure to consult your physician before starting the program. This is especially true for anyone who has not trained in a while. If you are worried about the possible effects on any old injury you might be nursing or any existing medical conditions, obtain an expert's opinion first and put your mind at rest. Physiotherapists and personal trainers experienced in injury rehabilitation will be able to evaluate any exercise and see possible warning signs to prevent damage. Sometimes just a small modification to a movement might be all that's needed to make it safe for you and help you obtain the full benefit of your training program.

Your mental attitude will make a big difference in the success of any training program. Worries about hurting yourself will hold you back from achieving the results that are possible with the training routines in this book.

How Will This Book Benefit Me?

These simple but powerful explanations and practical applications will make it easy to assess your unique fitness needs and design an exercise routine to suit any requirements. The versatility of resistance bands makes them an ideal exercise tool. They are lightweight and compact, making them easy to transport. They can be used in- or outdoors, at home or on vacation.

You will learn about the various types of tubing and bands available and how to choose the ideal one for you. You will also learn how to use the equipment correctly to prevent strain injuries, stay toned and fit, keep blood pressure normal, and aid in the healing of any existing injuries or post medical procedures.

Armed with information about the different body types, you will be able to put together a set of exercises tailored for your age, fitness level, and specific training for an activity or sport.

Who Is the Author?

Francis Papun is an ardent fitness enthusiast and coach who has helped individuals the last two decades take back control over their health and fitness. He is passionate about helping people build perfect bodies and healthier minds.

He believes in continual development and strives to assist people who want to achieve their happiest lives. Inspiring the youth to devote enough time to nurture healthy, strong bodies is also an important belief. He has a genuine desire to help others and knows success is only possible through dedication and hard work.

An author of a variety of health and fitness topics, Francis's aim is to help the reader understand staying fit and agile is not as hard as it seems. His books explain the secrets to making the necessary lifestyle changes that will transform body and mind. He leverages health and fitness training to polish and hone all the key attributes of people who struggle to keep up with a fast-moving world.

Francis is an expert at building robust fitness plans and aims to amalgamate his extensive knowledge and passion for fitness to help his readers to build perfect versions of themselves.

Besides this, Francis Papun remains an avid seeker of knowledge. He is always on the lookout for something new to learn, as well as staying alert to every opportunity to make a positive difference in someone's life.

He cherishes his family and friends and loves spending time with them.

Benefits of Regular Exercise for Seniors

A moving body is a healthy body, even well into old age. Regular exercise of the right kind has numerous benefits.

Prevention of Disease

Heart disease, hypertension, and diabetes have become part of our daily existence, and some people believe that contracting these illnesses in advanced years is unavoidable.

Regular exercise, however, strengthens the heart muscle, lowers blood pressure, and raises the levels of good cholesterol. This brings about better blood flow throughout the body and ensures more efficient heart activity ("Health Benefits Of Physical Activity," 2019).

Weight Management

Excess weight is a well-known risk factor in many diseases. Regular exercise increases the body's ability to burn calories and builds muscle mass for a stronger, healthier body.

Pain Management

Back pain is a common complaint among seniors. If it is caused by weak muscles that can no longer properly support the bone structure, regular exercise targeted at the right muscle groups will improve posture and add flexibility, thereby preventing or lessening back pain ("Health Benefits Of Physical Activity," 2019).

Bone Health

The condition of osteoporosis refers to fragile bones. When the formation of new bone cannot keep up with the loss of the old tissue, the bone structure becomes stressed. This weakens them to the point where even mild accidents can cause bone fractures. Regular strengthening exercises can prevent this from happening and minimize risk in older people. Women are especially prone to osteoporosis after menopause (Mayo Clinic, 2016).

Stress Reduction

Many studies have shown that physical exercise leads to an increase in mood-regulating chemicals (Collins, 2012). Movement stimulates inactive parts of the brain and neurotransmitters such as dopamine, serotonin, and endorphins are released. That also helps to maintain a balance with stress hormones such as adrenalin.

Prevention of Disability

Flexible, strong joints and muscles are an excellent defense against falls or accidents. It lowers the risk of serious injury and consequent disability significantly.

Maintaining Cognitive Function

Regular exercise has been shown to lower the risk of dementia by about 30 percent. Some studies suggest the risk for specifically Alzheimer's disease could even be halved when an exercise routine is started in later life (Alzheimer's Society UK, n.d.).

Social Engagement

A regular workout routine shared with others can provide essential social contact for seniors. Feelings of loneliness won't stand a chance, and exercising will never feel like a chore again.

My Promise to You

If you apply the easy principles explained in this book and invest time in compiling and regularly performing a set of resistance band exercises tailored to your needs, guided by the detailed information in this book, your body will yield years of interest on your investment.

You will experience far greater flexibility and fitness, as well as a much higher level of health than your peers who opted for inactivity. You will have the opportunity to prevent or improve some serious and debilitating illnesses.

The benefits are long-lasting because each exercise routine can easily be adjusted according to evolving needs. With portable and lightweight equipment like resistance bands, exercise can carry on well into advanced age.

But...You Have to Act!

There is no better time than the present to take control of your health and quality of life. You have all the tools you need in your hands with this book, regardless of your current age. Stop merely surviving and start thriving. Let's get started!

Chapter 1:

What is Resistance Training?

According to its definition, resistance, or strength training is described as activities of any kind that make muscles stronger (Merriam-Webster, 2011).

When thinking about resistance training, the first image that's likely to pop into your head is of burly muscled athletes lifting weights and barbells. It does not have to be that way though. This type of training can be done with the aid of simple tools, or bodyweight alone can be used to provide resistance. Its effectiveness lies in the fact that it builds muscle strength and endurance.

How Exactly Does the Body Build Muscle?

The easiest way to explain the process is to think about damage and subsequent repair happening within the body. Skeletal muscles are some of the most adaptable tissue in the body, and they always strive to repair any injury to fibers as soon as possible. This is done by rebuilding the injured muscle through satellite cells, which fuse and adhere to the muscle fibers. This enlarges the muscle and is known as cell hypertrophy (Kwon & Kravitz, 2019).

It is necessary to understand the word injury in a broader sense. Exercising a muscle and challenging it to its limits with an activity like resistance training causes trauma to the fibers inside the muscle. This trauma is referred to as injury in scientific terms, although it does not necessarily involve pain in the traditional sense of the word (Kwon & Kravitz, 2019). It is also called micro-trauma (Creveling, 2020).

The newly added satellite cells provide additional growth nuclei to the muscle, which enables the muscle to synthesize more protein than before and also utilize these building blocks more effectively than before.

One of the biggest advantages of using body weight as resistance is that no unnecessary load is added (Creveling, 2020). That yields the biggest gains in strength and flexibility for everyday activities with the least damage done. A win-win situation!

Studies have also shown regular resistance exercise to increase the protecting tissue network around muscles, thereby reducing the risk of injury even more (Kwon & Kravitz, 2019).

Other ways to build strength are:

- Pull-ups
- Squats
- Push-ups
- Planking
- Burpees
- Tricep dips
- Crawls
- Mountain climbers
- Box jumps

None of these methods involve any weights.

Why Are Bands a Good Choice?

There are several reasons why resistance bands or resistance tubing are a good choice for seniors (Lori Michiel Fitness, Inc, n.d.). Resistance bands are small and easily folded into a compact space. That means they travel well and suit any lifestyle. The durable material means it can be used indoors and outdoors. All levels of fitness can benefit from this type of training. While some super athletes regularly include resistance training with bands in their routines, it works equally well for someone just starting out with a new program or recovering from an injury. No gravity pull is involved like with weights, making it a very safe form of exercise. Because the body has to be stabilized all the time to counter the tension while using resistance bands, it greatly enhances coordination and balance.

Bands can be used to perform new and basic moves, or they can be incorporated into an existing routine to add variety and intensity. Just by positioning your body relative to the band differently, a new group of muscles can be targeted with the same exercise (Lori Michiel Fitness, Inc, n.d.).

Bands can be purchased in different strengths, as well as different forms and sizes. There are flat models or those rounded with handles also known as tubing. Many of them are color-coded according to various tension levels from easy to very heavy. Pink and yellow generally mean light tension, green and red moderate, and dark gray and black are considered intense. Generally, resistance bands are cheaply priced, especially if you want to purchase only one first to get started and see if it works for you. They can be purchased in stores or online.

No specialized equipment or installation is necessary to reap the full benefits of resistance band training. They can be looped around the body or anchored to a chair or table, or simply be pinned to the floor by hands or feet.

Making the Right Choice

A good way to start is by buying a set of three or four coordinated mini-bands with different resistance levels. The standard circumference is between 18 and 24 inches.

Add a pull-up assistance band to assist with movement without having to use full body weight. This type of band is longer than the mini-bands and should be strong enough to withstand all the bodyweight of the individual using it.

Look for bands that are comfortable to use. Padded, permanent handles usually feel more comfortable than detachable plastic handles.

Make sure the equipment you buy has all the accessories needed to make it fully functional. And always check with your doctor first if you have any existing condition or injury.

The Top 10 Resistance Band Training Rules

As with any activity, following simple rules for your safety and comfort is the best way to make the most out of your training sessions and achieve lasting results.

- **Always warm-up and stretch**

Before beginning any exercise routine, it is extremely important to warm the muscles and joints slowly up first. This will also ensure heart rate and body temperature don't spike but build up gradually to a level where exercise can be performed safely.

At the end of the program, the body has to be stretched gently to cool down. That will give the cardiovascular system a chance to return to resting levels in a controlled way (*The Right Way to Warm Up and Cool Down*, 2019).

In one of the later chapters, we'll delve deeper into dynamic warm-ups and stretching exercises.

- **Start with 30-minute sessions**

It might be tempting to jump into your new exercise routine with so much gusto that you feel you could achieve everything within a month. However, that is setting yourself up for failure.

Start with a commitment of only 30 minutes at a time and increase the time slowly as your strength and fitness grow. Once you are well-conditioned, the sessions can be continued up to 90 minutes.

- **Build a habit**

Muscle strength builds slowly, but it will only happen if training happens regularly. Sporadic training will decrease endurance and motivation, while the risk for injury is increased (YMCA of the North, n.d.).

- **Increase repetitions gradually**

A good number of repetitions to start with is eight. Gradually increase this to 15 and listen to your body to determine how quickly this can be done (Fitness Australia, 2018).

- **Aim for at least ten exercises**

Try to include ten exercises in your routine. Four of these should be for your lower body and six for the upper body. This should add enough variety to keep things interesting.

- **Perform movements in a controlled fashion**

Less really is more for seniors in terms of gains from exercise when controlled movements are used instead of power and momentum. A fast, strong movement targets different muscles than a slower, controlled one.

With the goals of balance and flexibility in mind, the muscles that control movement are the ones that should be exercised (Crowley, 2016).

- **Work larger muscles first**

As a general rule, larger muscles are exercised before smaller muscles (Jay, 2010). That means, for instance, working chest muscles first before getting to the shoulders. More difficult exercises will come before easier ones.

- **Perform a complete range of motion**

Performing the complete range of motion that a muscle is capable of, is the best way to exercise the whole muscle. This is especially important in the case of seniors, where regaining flexibility and mobility is vital. Using the full range of capabilities of a specific muscle will alleviate stiffness and pain caused by limited movements (Fetters, 2016).

It should be a pain-free movement, continuing as far as the joint will allow. Adjust the amount of resistance to accommodate a full range of motion.

- **Never hold your breath**

Correct breathing is very important and will be discussed in a later chapter. It is easy when concentrating on movement or form to hold your breath, as counterintuitive as that may sound.

Because our bodies are smart, our brains know when muscles need more oxygen. Oxygen is delivered in blood, so the heart rate increases to meet the higher demand. Holding your breath can cause your blood pressure to rise, due to the lack of adequate oxygen. This will achieve exactly the opposite result of what you want (Alexander, 2011). Instead, use the rhythm of exercise to learn deep and calm breathing.

- **Maintain the correct body alignment**

Body alignment or exercise posture refers to the relative positions of different body parts to each other during an exercise. Ignoring this can lead to injury or aggravate an existing condition.

General guidelines to keep in mind are (National Posture Institute, 2014):

- The head should be kept in line with the spine as far as possible, positioning the ears over the shoulders.
- The chin should be in line with the neck.
- The back should be straight, and the shoulders relaxed.
- The knees should not be locked.
- The pelvis should be tucked in somewhat, with the belly button pushing towards the spine.

When progressing too quickly to a more difficult exercise or higher resistance before the body is ready, muscles and joints will compensate for their difficulty in performing the movement by going out of alignment. That can put your whole exercise routine on hold for quite a while and cause unnecessary pain and discomfort.

The Bottom Line

Are you excited yet about the new you that is only one resistance band away? Seriously, the benefits of resistance band training almost speak for themselves.

Let's summarize the main takeaways of this chapter:

- Resistance training does not automatically equal extra weights. Although weightlifting is probably the best-known form of strength exercise, the same results can be achieved with resistance bands only.
- Strength training works because of the way our bodies build new muscle.
- Resistance bands are an excellent choice for seniors specifically because they are versatile, portable, light, cheap, easily obtainable, easy to use, and they enhance coordination, flexibility, and balance more than other types of strength training.
- If you follow the ten rules of resistance band training and you have the go-ahead from your

physician, it is one of the safest forms of exercise possible for seniors. Just to recap:
- Always do warm-ups before and stretches after exercising.
- Stick to half an hour sessions for a start.
- Make it a habit.
- Increase repetitions gradually.
- Work up to ten exercises per session.
- Control movements.
- Work on larger muscles first.
- Perform the full range of motion a muscle can do.
- Breathe!
- Keep proper body alignment.

In only a few weeks' time, you will feel supercharged and people will start to notice your confidence and radiance.

So get started today, why wait?

Chapter 2:

Healing From Injury

Training with resistance bands to recuperate from an injury is an excellent way to strengthen the muscles again after a period of inactivity.

As with any exercise activity, seniors should keep a few things in mind when embarking on this healing journey to make it effective and prevent aggravation of the injury.

Common Injuries Healed With Resistance Training

Resistance bands are the ideal aids to focus on the muscle or group of damaged muscles because the maximum amount of stress can be put on the muscle without straining the joint unduly (*Rehabbing Sports Injuries with Resistance Bands*, 2018).

Shoulder Dislocation or Pain

According to a study done by the American Academy of Orthopaedic Surgeons, about one-fifth of all shoulder dislocations occur in patients older than 60 years. These patients are also more likely to suffer injury to the rotator cuff during dislocation because the tissue surrounding the cuff gets weaker with age (Murthi & Ramirez, 2012).

Older populations the world over are more active for longer than a few decades ago, and injuries can occur easily.

Other signs to watch for without actual dislocation having taken place are tingling or numbness, significant weakening of the hand and arm when compared to the other side, and persistent and unexplained pain or tenderness in the area.

Tennis Elbow

Contrary to popular belief, tennis elbow does not only come from prolonged tennis play. Any repetitive motion that damages the tendons connecting the forearm to the elbow can cause pain in the outer part of the elbow.

Activities such as gardening, painting, using a screwdriver, or even knitting or crocheting can be the source of the damage. The main concept here is overuse (Healthwise Incorporated, 2020).

Any rehab exercises should aim to lengthen the tendons again and strengthen them.

Runner's Knee

Another slight misnomer, the condition does not refer to a specific injury. It is a term that is used to indicate a broad range of knee problems, and the medical term is patellofemoral pain syndrome (WebMD, 2007).

It can be caused by any repetitive movement, for which the knee is not strong enough like stepping up the number of repetitions in an exercise routine too soon, or by a fall or other direct hit to the kneecap. Misalignment between hips and ankles or thigh muscles that are too weak to keep the kneecap in its proper place during movement could also cause pain, as can any foot problems common in the elderly (WebMD, 2007).

Hip Bursitis

Large joints like hips have fluid-filled sacs called bursae next to them to lubricate movement and protect the bone. If a bursae becomes inflamed for any reason, the condition is called bursitis.

Overuse, injury, or complications after hip surgery can cause it. Poor posture and weak muscles could predispose a person to develop bursitis (WebMD, n.d.).

Sprains and Strains

These two types of injuries have proved to be the nemesis of many older athletes. A resistance band workout offers a safe way to build strength again slowly.

A sprain occurs when a ligament is overstretched or overworked, while a strain refers to the same mechanism injuring a muscle or tendon (Giacobbe, 2019).

As soon as the injury has healed enough to allow for exercising, resistance bands for easy stretching can be used to gradually get moving again. As strength returns, bands with higher tension can be introduced until the ligament, muscle or tendon is back to the pre-injury level.

Recovery After Knee-Repair Surgery

This type of surgery is usually performed to repair the anterior cruciate ligaments or ACL. These ligaments hold the knee together and can get injured by a movement as simple as getting out of a car and turning too quickly to another direction.

In older people, the injury is often associated with weakened hamstrings (Quinn, 2020). Resistance band exercises present the perfect opportunity to strengthen and lengthen the hamstrings again gradually while also strengthening the knee and surrounding ligaments themselves.

Phases of Recuperation After Injury

Understanding the general phases of recovery can be very helpful in designing the right post-injury exercise routine. Three stadia can be identified as (New Heights Physical Therapy, n.d.):

- Reaction
- Regeneration
- Remodeling

Reaction Phase

The first 24 to 72 hours after sustaining an injury, the body responds to the trauma with swelling and muscle spasms among other things. Movement is painful and the natural reaction to this is to take painkillers and immobilize the injured part of the body.

A small, controlled amount of movement is necessary, however, to aid in the flushing of waste products and bringing in much-needed oxygen and nutrients to prevent the formation of scar tissue and start the healing process (New Heights Physical Therapy, n.d.).

Regeneration

The formation of new tissue and the repair of any damaged nerve connections starts next and takes anywhere between six and eight weeks (New Heights Physical Therapy, n.d.).

The aim of any physical exercise during this period is to minimize pain while maximizing the generation and strengthening of new tissue. One of the ways to do this is to gently increase the range of motion in a controlled manner.

Remodeling Stage

This is the final stage to complete recovery and can take between three months to a year. Although acute pain might be something of the past by now, it is still extremely important to manage the exercise routine correctly to prevent chronic pain from developing.

The focus should be on strengthening supporting tissue, muscles, and ligaments because the area is vulnerable and there is a danger of recurring injury (New Heights Physical Therapy, n.d.).

A Note of Caution

No workout should be started without consulting your physician first, especially not when recovering from an injury.

Be cautious if you:

- Have any shortness of breath without exertion.
- Have chest pains or pain in your left arm and neck.
- Take medication for high blood pressure.
- Have arthritis.
- Have osteoporosis.
- Have dizzy spells.
- Are extremely overweight.
- Have diabetes.

Always make sure you listen to your body. A good rule of thumb to follow is the "talk test." You should be able to talk normally while exercising. If you get out of breath, it is time to take it slower (Schrift, 2014).

Breathe, Breathe, Breathe…

Breathing is one of those automatic, instinctive actions needed for our survival, and it might sound strange to be reminded to do it. Many people, however, when they exercise, forget to breathe or breathe incorrectly during a movement.

Muscles use more oxygen when contracting than when resting, and the only way to deliver the much-needed element is by breathing deeply in the right pattern.

In and Out

The simplest breathing technique is to breathe in on a contraction and out on an extension (Taraniuk, 2019).

Let's illustrate that with some easy exercises:

- Squat: Breathe in while lowering your body into a squatting position (contraction). Breathe out while straightening your legs to a standing position again (extension).
- Chest press: Exhale as you push the resistance band handles away from you, inhale as you bring your hands back toward your chest.
- Glute bridge: Exhale when lifting your hips off the floor and inhale when lowering them again.

Women with flexible bands, ready to do a chest press

Belly Breathing

It is deeper than chest breathing and is also called diaphragmatic breathing. When you pull air in through your nose and feel your belly puffing up, you are using your diaphragm.

Benefits of belly breathing include lowering of heart rate and blood pressure, as well as enhancing the body's capacity for enduring exercise (Jewell, 2018).

A good way to teach yourself belly breathing is to concentrate on a sequence of breathing in for three counts and breathing out for two (Newhouse, 2013). If you do this while going about everyday activities, it will be second nature when you start your workout routine.

Consistency Is Key

Whether you do your workout three times a week or five times a week, being consistent matters more than the type of exercises or number of repetitions in terms of measurable results.

In a recent study undertaken by the University of New South Wales in Sydney's School of Medical Sciences, lead author Mandy Hagstrom found consistent and frequent exercise to be some of the key factors in a successful resistance training program (Hagstrom et al., 2019).

It is therefore important to set realistic goals for yourself. Design your workout to fit into your daily and monthly schedule. Make allowances for any illnesses or physical weaknesses you might have. Unrealistic goals lead to unrealistic expectations, which set you up for failure before you've even started.

Your health and well-being are far too important to sabotage your success by aiming too high.

The Role of Genetics

Our genes are the inescapable blueprints of who we are. They determine everything, from hair and eye color to personality.

Genes also determine body type, which influences how easy or difficult it is to get fit and flexible. But being inescapable does not equal the end of workout plans if your body type, it just means you may have to work a bit smarter to gain the same results as someone else.

The concept of different general body types has been around since the time of Plato. In the 1940s, American psychologist William Sheldon popularized three categories here (Snape, 2015) and identified them as ectomorph, endomorph, and mesomorph.

Each type has to train differently from the others, because muscle composition, among other factors, seems to vary.

Ectomorphs

This body type, especially among women, is very envied in modern times because they are skinny, long-limbed people who never seem to gain weight. They have fast metabolisms that rapidly convert sugars into energy.

This is not without problems though, because they have to work much harder to gain muscle mass through exercise. This has consequences in later years when muscle mass starts decreasing with age, and an exercise routine for a senior ectomorph will look different from any of the others.

Endomorphs

These are the bigger, pear-shaped people with shorter limbs and broader hips. They tend to put on weight easily. Unfortunately, a lot of this weight is fat and not muscle. They often have the hardest time getting fit and toned, but it is definitely attainable.

Ectomorphs

This group seems to fall in the middle of the first two. They don't store fat as easily and don't find it too hard to build muscle.

They are often referred to as "naturally athletic," and chances are that fitness was neglected in their younger days because they did not seem to need to workout.

The later years bring their own challenges with diminishing muscle mass and declining mobility, so this body type can benefit just as much from a regular resistance band routine as any of the others.

Types of Resistance Bands

There are six types of bands, and some have very specific uses. They are mini bands (also known as fit loop bands), tubing, therapy bands, figure 8 bands, ring bands, and lateral resistance bands.

The first two are the most versatile for general purposes (*The Definitive Guide to Resistance Bands and Workout Bands*, n.d.).

Mini Bands

They are flat with no handles and form a continuous loop. They are generally four inches to two feet long, and although they work well to train the lower body, any muscle group can be targeted depending on the size of the band. They are ideal for reaching muscles that would otherwise be difficult to isolate.

Mini bands come in different widths, from paper-thin to thick, and can be made from a variety of materials. Latex is the most common type, but for those with a latex allergy, there are fabric and elastic types.

If you plan on buying only one type of band to start, mini bands are a good option. Go for a thicker version to allow for a wide scope of exercises.

A set of mini bands.

Tubing

These are tubular rather than flat as the title suggests, open-ended, and have handles at the ends. With an average length of around four feet, they are mostly used to strengthen the upper body.

Tubular bands are commonly found in gyms, personal training studios, and outdoor boot camps. Some have hooks attached to the ends so that different bands can be hooked together or other accessories can be attached.

Tubular resistance band with handles.

The Resistance Level

The intensity of a workout depends on the thickness of the band, as well as how far it is stretched. As you get stronger, you might decide not to change your exercises, but only to change the resistance before moving on to another exercise all together.

How to Find the Right Level

The appropriate resistance level at any given time depends on the exercise and the number of repetitions you're aiming for.

Start with the band offering the least resistance. The average number of repetitions should be between 10 and 15 for every exercise. You should feel challenged by about the seventh repetition. If you can do all the repetitions with this band without feeling tired, you should move up to the next band level (Kassel, 2019).

On the other hand, if you get the feeling during an exercise that you can't control the band, as if your arm or leg is about to be snapped back, then the resistance level is too high. Performing an exercise that way puts your body at risk of going out of alignment, which can be detrimental in the long run.

Adjusting Resistance During an Exercise

It is quick and simple to adjust on the go because resistance bands are so versatile.

You could either add bands, adjust your position or the position of the band.

- Adding bands to the one already in use will immediately increase the resistance experienced and make the exercise harder.
- Resistance is also influenced by the distance you stand from an anchor point in exercises that require anchors. For a standing row exercise, for example, the band needs to be looped around or fastened to an immovable object. Standing closer to the anchor point will make the exercise easier while moving away will make it harder.

- The resistance will change from a band looped above your knees to around your shins, then ankles.

Do You Need More Convincing?

If you're still wondering if resistance bands will work for you, let's look at the benefits again. The great thing is, these benefits will be accurate for you regardless of your age or fitness level (8fit Team, n.d.).

Resistance band workouts force muscles to contract when the band is stretched, which tones and strengthens. It is a controllable and gentle way for older people to achieve results. Resistance bands can also be used to assist in exercise. If a pull up for instance looks impossible to do, use a band attached to the bar to make it easier until you can perform it unassisted.

Nobody likes aching muscles, rigid and tight with tension. Use resistance bands to gently stretch back, shoulder, and neck muscles to remove the caught-up tension and find natural pain relief.

Your resistance bands will travel wherever you go. They're light and easy to fold, taking up very little space in a suitcase. As far as training equipment goes, this is one of the most affordable options available. The grandkids might even enjoy exercising with you!

Resistance bands don't need gravity to do their job like weights, which make them easier on joints and muscles that are not so young anymore. A wider range of motion is possible, which means better flexibility and strengthening can be achieved. Many exercises can be done in a sitting position, making an exercise routine accessible to people who might normally have been excluded.

Not only muscles but bones and joints benefit from resistance band workouts. Strength training stimulates bones to make new cells, keeping osteoporosis at bay and decreasing the likelihood of broken bones if a small tumble should happen.

The low impact of resistance band exercises is very kind to joints as well. They are also ideal for recovering after an injury when exercise should be targeted but gentle.

Before we start with the nitty-gritty of an exercise routine in the next chapters, this could be a good time to go back over the previous chapters and make sure you know and understand everything involved.

You can always refer back to this outline, and you might even pick something up that you missed the first time.

Are you ready to start warming up?

Chapter 3:

Warm-Ups and Stretches

You wouldn't expect to be able to reach down to the floor and touch your toes first thing in the morning after getting out of bed stiffly and cautiously. Equally, you can't expect your body to perform exercise routines without having been prepared first.

Not only will muscles and joints be endangered if a proper warm-up is neglected, but to burst into sudden vigorous activity can overwork the heart. Warming up gradually speeds up the heart and breathing gradually, which delivers more blood and oxygen to the muscles and prepares them for more intense activity.

The reverse is true at the end of the workout if movement comes to a stop without gently slowing down with stretches. A cooling down stretching routine brings everything back to resting tempo with no sudden changes.

Furthermore, easing into your workout with warm-ups puts you in the right frame of mind to make the most of your active time.

Suggested Exercises

Let's look at a couple of warm-up exercises and stretches in practical detail.

Windmill Exercise

This exercise loosens the shoulders but is also very beneficial for core strength and overall stability (Fetters, 2019).

- Start by standing with your feet slightly wider than hip-width. Turn your left foot out at an angle of 90 degrees and raise your right arm to the ceiling while looking up at your right hand.
- Slide your left arm down your left leg as far as possible without putting any pressure on the leg. Bend the leg slightly to avoid locking the knee.
- Move your hips slightly to your right and use your core to stabilize yourself while sliding your left arm down.
- Pause at the lowest point for a couple of seconds before pushing yourself upright again. Keep your spine straight all the time.
- Do five to eight repetitions before switching sides.

Elbow Touch

This exercise is beneficial to the chest, shoulders, and rotator cuff.

- Sit or stand with proper body alignment and place your right hand on your right shoulder and your left hand on your left shoulder.
- Move your arms towards each other until your elbows touch.
- Move your elbows out to the sides while attempting to squeeze your shoulder blades closer to each other.
- Visualize your chest opening up and stretching to admit more oxygen.
- Return your elbows to the starting position in a controlled movement.
- Do five to eight repetitions.

Tennis Elbow Warm-Up

If you are exercising to help heal a tennis elbow, it is especially important to warm the elbow and surrounding muscles and tendons up first to avoid increasing pain.

- Sit at a table with your arm comfortably stretched out on the table, palm facing up.

- Touch every finger to your thumb, starting with the pinkie.
- Do five to eight repetitions before switching sides.

Shoulder Box Exercise

The target of this exercise is the trapezius muscle. It is a large triangular muscle in the upper back that stretches the whole width between the shoulders. It reaches down to the thoracic part of the spine (De Pietro, 2019).

The trapezius plays a big role in shoulder and neck mobility and helps to stabilize the shoulders during some arm movements.

Pain in this area is often caused by stress, overuse, or poor posture, such as sitting hunched over a computer all day.

- Tie your resistance band to a solid anchoring object at your shoulder height.
- Hold your arms straight out in front of you, level with your shoulders.
- Keep a little bit of tension in the band so that your chest pulls forward slightly.
- Move your arms out to the sides with the backs of your hands facing up.

- Squeeze your shoulders together for a couple of seconds before returning to the starting position slowly.
- Do five to eight repetitions (Mirafit, n.d.).

A variation without the resistance band can be done by standing comfortably with your arms hanging by your sides.

- While inhaling through the nose, slowly pull your shoulders up towards your ears, as far as is comfortable for you.
- Pull your shoulder blades back towards each other, and push your shoulders down at the same time.
- Hold for a couple of seconds before slowly returning to the starting position (Knopf, 2010).

Choker Exercise

The shoulders and rotator cuff are sometimes difficult to isolate and reach. This exercise is excellent for doing just that and is a great pain reliever when stress is the culprit.

- Sit or stand with your right hand on your left shoulder.
- Place your left hand under your right elbow and gently push your right arm upwards towards

your throat so that your elbow stops in line with your nose.
- Hold for 10 seconds and release.
- Do five to eight repetitions and switch sides (Knopf, 2010).

A variation on this exercise for even more stretch is to take your right hand off your shoulder and straighten the arm when it reaches the top position.

Wrist Stretch

If you are a constant computer or smartphone user, your wrists will need special attention with a couple different stretches.

- Stretch your arm out in front of you with the palm turned up towards the ceiling.
- Bend your wrist down as far as possible so that your fingers point towards the floor.
- Take hold of your fingers with your other hand and gently pull them towards your body until you can feel a stretch in the underside of your wrist.
- Hold for a couple of seconds and relax.
- Repeat five to eight times.

Stretch the top of your wrist as well by doing the same exercise, only keep your palm facing the floor (Fort Healthcare, 2019).

Knee to Chest Exercise

The lower back and gluteus maximus (or glute for short) are often problem areas in older people. Glutes are the main hip muscles and are connected to the lower back and thighs. Spasms in this muscle can make it painful to stand up or sit down.

A comfortable and safe way to perform the knee to chest stretch is to do it in a prone position.

- Lie down fully stretched out on your back.
- Bring one knee up to your chest and wrap your arms around your leg below the knee.
- Pull the knee closer gently as far as is comfortable and hold for a couple of seconds.
- Lower the leg and do the same stretch with the other one.
- Repeat five to eight times.

If your back is strong enough, you could lift both knees at the same time (Kendola, 2020).

Sit & Reach Exercise

The next body parts to receive attention are the hamstrings. They are often shortened, stiff, and painful in seniors because of decreased mobility.

The sit and reach exercise is commonly used by fitness coaches to determine a person's flexibility and assess their risk for future injury.

- If it is possible for you, sit flat on the floor near a wall or other flat object, with your legs stretched out in front of you.
- Keep your knees straight and make sure feet are up against the wall while you remain flat on the floor.
- Bend forward and stretch your arms out as far as they can go.
- Keep the position for a couple of seconds.
- Repeat five times if possible (Quinn, 2008).

If you cannot sit on the floor, you can perform the exercise on a chair.

- Sit forward on the seat with one leg stretched out straight in front of you.
- Tilt the foot of the outstretched leg up.
- Bend forward, keeping your body in a straight line, and reach down with your hand towards your foot, as far as you can go.

Rear Calf Stretch Exercise

Tight or painful calves can hamper movement significantly. For the elderly, poor circulation is often to blame for this condition. This stretch can go a long way to alleviate the discomfort.

- Stand while holding on to the back of a chair with one foot in front of the other.
- Bend the knee of the front foot slightly.
- Lean forward towards the chair while keeping the back leg completely straight (Marcin, 2018).

Gas Pedal Exercise

Ankles are vulnerable and easy to injure when flexibility lessens, and movement becomes more difficult. It is, therefore, imperative to look after ankle health and make sure they are properly warmed up and stretched.

The gas pedal stretch is done with the aid of a resistance band.

- Sit on a chair with one leg stretched out in front of you and your back kept straight.
- Loop the band under the outstretched foot where the instep is.
- Pull the band up tight enough that you can feel tension around your foot.

- Push your foot down against the band as if you are using the gas pedal of a car.
- Repeat five to eight times and change feet (University Orthopedics, n.d.).

Twister Exercise

The torso twist is a great way to warm up your core muscles and enhance flexibility at the same time. A word of caution if you are prone to dizzy spells: take it slowly and carefully.

- Stand with your feet shoulder-width apart.
- Bend your elbows so your arms form a 90-degree angle.
- Swing your shoulders and torso from one side to the other.
- Look in the direction where you are moving and pivot your feet with the movement.
- Allow your right heel to lift when twisting to the left and the left heel to lift when twisting to the right.
- Keep your head up, and your neck relaxed.
- Remember to control the movement; don't jerk or try to do it too fast (Pedemonte, 2020).

Side Bend Exercise

Another good movement to benefit the torso and shoulders is the side bend.

- Stand with your feet comfortably placed about shoulder-width apart.
- Keep your back straight and bend down to one side, reaching with that hand towards the floor.
- Hold the stretch for a couple of seconds and come up slowly.
- Do the same to the other side.
- Remember to control the movement at all times so as not to compromise the spine (Winderl, 2017).

Rock 'n Roll Exercise

A slow, gentle version of rocking and rolling can do wonders for any tight or sore lower back area while strengthening the torso and core muscles.

- Lie down on your back on the floor.
- Pull your knees up and keep your feet flat on the ground.
- Roll your knees slowly and gently to one side and then to the other.
- Make sure your shoulders stay firmly on the ground and don't move with your lower body.

- Repeat five to eight times (Cadman, 2020).

Head Lift Exercise

A stiff and painful neck is, unfortunately, one of the realities of our modern, stressful life. It is also a vulnerable part of the body and should be warmed up gently to prevent injury.

- Go down on your hands and knees and keep your body in alignment with hands under shoulders and knees under hips.
- Keep your back straight and drop your head slowly down towards your chest.
- Tuck in your chin and hold the position for five seconds.
- Then raise your head again slowly to be level with your back.
- Do five to eight repetitions.
- Remember to keep the movement controlled at all times (Fairview, n.d.).

Tennis Watcher Exercise

Another one for the neck is done seated.

- Inhale through your nose and look towards your left as far as you can comfortably turn your head.
- Hold the position for a few seconds.
- Exhale through your mouth, and slowly turn your head back to face forwards again.
- Repeat the process to the other side.
- Keep the movement slow and controlled.
- Do five to eight repetitions (Dotfit, n.d.).

Chapter 4:

Understanding the Benefits of Strength Training

Every journey has to start somewhere. Deciding to exercise towards a healthier, fitter, and happier you is no exception.

You might have tried in the past only to be turned around or mitigated some of the negative consequences of getting older. Anything new can be scary and uncomfortable at first, especially if you are not fully convinced you will make a difference.

If you are still on the fence about strength training, I want to tell you a bit more about this concept and its benefits for you. I understand your hesitation and would like to show you where this can lead if you allow it to keep building momentum.

Strength Training in a Nutshell

Strength or resistance training helps muscles and joints remain fully functional at any age, and preserves mobility well into the golden years. Strong, flexible muscles and joints make daily activities much easier and contribute to general happiness and a feeling of well-being. Workouts can be adapted to all fitness levels, and most existing chronic diseases can be managed and even improved through regular resistance training sessions (Mayo Clinic, 2018). Let's break this down into more bite-size chunks.

From the age of 30, we start losing muscle mass to the tune of three to five percent per year (Iliades, 2019). Strength workouts can be designed with exercises that target specific muscles or muscle groups, making them stronger and stimulating them to form new tissue.

If a muscle has a problem already like the back, strengthening the muscles around the problem area minimizes pain and discomfort and makes movement easier. Stronger muscles protect the joints around which they are, so the joints can keep functioning the way they should (Iliades, 2019).

Exercise stimulates the cells that form new bone. That will prevent osteoporosis, which is the weakening of bones mostly in older people. If there is osteoporosis already present, the condition will improve when bone density increases. The hips, spine, and wrists are prime candidates for osteoporosis and will benefit greatly from strength training (Wheeler, 2019).

Many seniors complain of struggling to keep their balance. Everyday things like climbing stairs become a nightmare, which has a limiting effect on their enjoyment of life. The balance problem stems from weakness in the hips, legs, ankles, and all the surrounding muscles. The right resistance exercises target these areas and restore strength. That decreases the likelihood of falls and fractures, which boosts self-confidence and quality of life (Wheeler, 2019).

A strength workout with resistance bands eliminates the need to visit a gym to gain access to equipment and personal trainers. You already have everything you need to make the most out of the bands in your home. With this book in your hands, there are no more excuses to get started.

Physical exercise is an instant mood boost. The exertion causes dopamine and other feel good neurotransmitters to be released in the brain, which brings feelings of happiness and a relaxed frame of mind. A regular resistance workout burns calories and helps to keep weight down. That lightens the load on joints and muscles, making the senior years much easier with regards to mobility.

Does grocery shopping leave you out of breath? A regular strength workout will improve endurance and stamina and life will definitely get easier. The added energy makes for a good night's sleep after an active day. Insomnia will also be something of the past (Mayo Clinic, 2018).

Strength Training and Diseases

Several chronic and acute conditions can improve or be prevented through regular resistance training.

- **Heart Disease**

Strength training has been shown to help in lowering blood pressure, and reducing the load on the heart. The risk of cardiac arrest decreases when the heart is not under so much strain. That contributes to peace of mind which lowers stress levels, making your heart's environment even stronger (Mayo Clinic, 2018).

- **Diabetes**

Regular exercise helps to regulate insulin that keeps blood sugar levels under control. Researchers have found that physical activity increases the effectiveness of the protein APPL1, which plays an integral role in the absorption of glucose (Upham, 2018).

- **Arthritis**

Resistance exercise can alleviate joint stiffness and lessen pain, because the surrounding muscles are getting stronger. That leads to a vastly improved quality of life for those with arthritis (Mayo Clinic, 2018).

- **Asthma**

The severity and frequency of asthma attacks can be positively influenced by regular exercise, because lung function and capacity improve with resistance training (Mayo Clinic, 2018).

- **Back Pain**

Much of the back pain older people suffer is due to weakness of the supporting muscles. Targeted resistance exercises strengthen them while improved flexibility minimizes the strain put on the spine during movement.

- **Cancer Recovery**

One of the most debilitating symptoms cancer survivors have to contend with is overwhelming fatigue and weakness. The gentle and adaptable nature of a resistance band workout helps with overall recovery to increase stamina according to the individual's physical condition.

- **Dementia**

Regular physical activity and the accompanying higher oxygen content in the blood can improve cognitive function in individuals with dementia (Mayo Clinic, 2018).

Increasing Anaerobic Endurance

Anaerobic exercises like resistance training use muscle energy without oxygen, as opposed to aerobic exercises that need a constant supply of oxygen (Kelly, 2015).

Examples of aerobic exercises are fast-paced activities like jogging or swimming. Anaerobic activities use slower, shorter bursts to access the glucose in muscles without using oxygen. This stimulates bone growth, increasing density, and keeping osteoporosis at bay. It also improves overall bodily strength and endurance, making daily life that much easier to negotiate. It also increases the body's ability to handle lactic acid, which in turn increases your stamina for workouts (Kelly, 2015).

The Cardiovascular and Pulmonary Systems

Our hearts and lungs are among the first organs to really show signs of wear and tear in later years. Strength training can help you turn the clock back somewhat, even when battling a pulmonary infection or heart condition.

As joints and muscles get weaker with age, it becomes harder to move the body. That makes the heart and lungs work much harder to do the same things as bef0re. A stronger body equals fewer aches and pains and more energy to enjoy life.

The lungs do not have to work so hard, because resistance training improves blood circulation and the available oxygen is utilized better.

As the circulatory system improves, metabolism speeds up and weight loss is kickstarted.

A Solution for the Whole Body

Resistance training offers a broad spectrum improvement package. Let's recap quickly.

- Muscles grow and become stronger, while joints are better protected and gain flexibility.
- Balance improves because muscles are stronger and joints move more easily.
- Pain is reduced because the body is stimulated into using its own healing mechanisms. A stronger frame that moves with less friction also limits everyday aches. Arthritis and lower back pain sufferers especially benefit from this.
- The heart, lungs, and circulatory system become more efficient.
- Bone density increases because bones are stimulated to grow. Studies have shown physical exercise activates cells called osteoblasts. This chemical signal encourages deposits of calcium and other minerals necessary for bone growth (Weingart & Kravitz, 2020).

An "Anti-Aging Formula"

A study at the University of Birmingham (2018) found that a group of older lifelong amateur athletes had not undergone as much muscle and bone loss as people of a similar age who never exercised. Their cholesterol levels were also lower than expected, and their immune systems were stronger than the control group. The men had essentially avoided most of male menopause with their testosterone levels measuring significantly higher than their inactive counterparts in age.

Studies like these disproved the assumption that age makes us frail and that it is unavoidable. It is never too late to start a workout program and reap benefits for years to come.

Factors Affecting Success

Your strength workout success can be outlined by a few things. All of these issues are within your control and you can decide whether they will stand in your way or not.

Nutrition

Your diet will greatly affect your results, whether your main goal is weight management, fitness, or both. A balanced intake of food will supply your body with all the calories and nutrients needed for everyday activities with a workout thrown in. It is not only the type of meal that is important though, but also the time of day when it is eaten (Kilroy, 2014).

- **Breakfast**

Breakfast really is important, because it is the first meal after many hours without any nutrient absorption.

Blood sugar levels are low and have to be restored to normal to supply fuel to your brain and body.

Protein plays an important role in this process. Simple and refined carbohydrates like a bagel on its own just won't cut it for long enough to get you through a workout without feeling lethargic and dizzy.

Instead, go for more complex carbohydrates with protein added like a slice of wholewheat toast with an egg or cheese. Avoid sugary cereals which can cause a blood sugar spike with a crash afterward, leaving you tired and feeling down. Rather go for oatmeal or wholegrain cereals with protein in the form of milk, yogurt or nuts added (Kilroy, 2014).

Carbohydrates supply more than half of our daily energy needs, despite the bed rap it has thanks to low carb diets. It should be complex carbs, however, which take longer to digest and keep us feeling full for longer. That is especially helpful in weight loss.

Examples of complex carbs are whole grain products, unprocessed foods, vegetables, fruits, and beans.

- **Snacks**

Your body needs food every two to four hours to keep blood sugar levels in the optimal range to supply energy for all activities, mental and physical.

Add a healthy snack to your diet mid morning and mid afternoon, especially before exercising. The ideal snack contains protein and vegetables or fruit in small portions (Level et al., 2017). It could be for example a small piece of cheese and an apple, or a whole grain snack cracker with a slice of cold chicken or turkey on top.

A small amount of healthy unsaturated fat is also recommended. Go for a drop of olive oil on your toast and leave the butter (Kilroy, 2014).

- **Main Meal**

Your main meal of the day can contain bigger portions of protein and carbohydrates than the other two meals, in addition to a healthy portion of vegetables. It should preferably not be eaten just before going to bed, as the energy used by your digestive system to convert the food could interfere with sleeping. That will rob you of a good night's rest and leave your body with nutrients that can't be used as they should, ending up being stored as fat.

If possible, the biggest meal of the day should be consumed in the afternoon before 15:00 for the best weight loss and fitness results (Kilroy, 2014).

- **Pre-Workout Snacks**

Enjoying a snack containing balanced amounts of protein and carbohydrates just before starting your workout can ensure sustained energy throughout. That will avoid any sudden drops in blood pressure and sugar levels and provide the optimal physical environment to set you up for success.

Good candidates on this snack list are bananas, berries, grapes, oranges, nuts, and nut butters.

Protein is not called the building blocks of life for nothing. Protein molecules are broken down by the body into smaller molecules called amino acids (HEB, 2020). Amino acids are indispensable for muscle and tissue growth and repair.

How to Avoid the Weight Loss Stall

We all know losing weight depends on taking in less calories than before, so that our bodies can start using the stored fat reserves instead of just using the new calories and storing even more.

Sometimes even a tight hold on the number of calories eaten with regular workouts doesn't have the desired result. Weight loss just plateaus and nothing seems to get it going again.

- An important factor in this equation is the amount of stress you are under. Stress causes the secretion of the hormone cortisol from the adrenal glands (Kamau, 2020). Cortisol changes the way the body uses nutrients and can cause

storage of energy as fat, instead of converting it into energy.
- Not getting enough slee[also changes your metabolic rate, which is the rate at which sugars are converted to energy (Kamau, 2020). Getting less uninterrupted sleep than what your body requires (on average about seven hours per night for adults) causes stress, which brings us back to the stress hormone cortisol. Most muscle growth also takes place during sleep, as well as repair to tissues. Strength training keeps on giving long after you finished your workout, working to build your new body while you rest.
- Water weight can be a contributing factor for seniors. Some medications cause water retention, as can eating too much salt and carbohydrates (Kamau, 2020).
- Once you start building muscle mass and bone density, your weight might also seem to stand still or even go up slightly. Don't be discouraged by this, you are winning the battle!

Body Composition

Your body consists of fat mass and fat-free mass. This is referred to as body composition (Tinsley, 2017).

Weight loss is affected by the changes in these two categories. If they change by the same amount at the same time, it stands to reason that no change in body weight will be detectable. For your resistance workout to be successful, you want the fat mass to decrease and the fat-free mass to increase. That is the formula for becoming the fitter, healthier and stronger you.

With the advice in this book you definitely are on the right road to achieving just that. It is within your reach to live a physically fulfilling and healthy life in your senior years. That will make it possible to stay independent for far longer and live life on your terms.

Chapter 5:

Types of Resistance Bands and Specifications

There are many variations of resistance bands available, and they can be confusing to a first time user.

Each type has its own advantages and disadvantages, and experience will teach you which ones, or which combinations will suit your needs. If you look after them well, clean them regularly, and keep plastic and latex away from UV light when possible, you should get a long life of happy exercising from them.

For general purposes, a set of loops and a set of tubes with all the different resistant levels will be a good starting point to attain general fitness. As you progress through your workout routines, you will need to increase resistance to keep your muscles developing, and it is easier when you have the necessary equipment at hand without having to go to the store first.

If your aim with the workouts is to rehabilitate after an injury, therapy bands are probably a good starting point.

They are gentle on weak muscles and long enough to be adequate for various exercise types.

The figure 8-band is versatile, and if you want to try with only one specialty band first on top of the basics, this is a dependent go-to for a wide variety of movements.

Attachments such as door anchors and ankle straps are nice to have but not essential in the beginning.

Do not worry; this chapter will provide a solid understanding of each type so you can make smart purchases and build your home gym to your advantage.

Loop Resistance Bands

Loop bands are exactly that - a continuous loop that is lightweight and versatile to use (Starwood Sports, n.d.). They are essentially big rubber bands. This type of band is popular to target and activate smaller groups of muscles that are sometimes overshadowed by their bigger neighbors and kept from getting a good workout.

Loop bands can also be added to others to change an exercise slightly or increase resistance. Exercises with loop bands can "wake up" muscles that have become lazy or strengthen stabilizing muscles to make movement safer.

This type of band comes in different colors, each with a different resistance level, although they are not available in ultra-heavy. Some core and upper body exercises are, therefore, not advisable with only loop bands (Simple Fitness Solutions, n.d.).

The same exercise can be done with all the different colors, increasing the intensity of the workout with every step up. They are also known as power bands.

They are available in different materials, from latex to rubber to material.

O-Shaped Expanders

Though these bands look like loops, they are generally shorter. They are good for lower body exercises. One disadvantage is that they tend to roll up around the ankles because they are fairly narrow, making them ineffective, and sometimes the skin gets pinched in the process (Simple Fitness Solutions, n.d.).

Tube Resistance Bands

The biggest difference between loops and tubes is that tubes are open-ended like skipping ropes, with handles. They can be made from thermoplastic or extruded rubber, or latex.

A tube with padded handles.

Some have detachable handles while the handles of others are fixed. Handles can be padded or just plain hard plastic.

Some are also manufactured with clips at the ends to hook a variety of accessories for different exercises.

They are often longer than flat bands at about four feet, and the excess length can make them difficult to use when doing exercises like chest presses. In movements where only one handle is used, the other one can also get in the way.

Tubes are also not recommended for leg exercises on isolated muscles, because longer flat bands or pull-up bands provide more room for movement. Multi-joint exercises do not present the same problem.

Tubing with handles makes exercises where two sides must be worked at the same time more simple. When no door anchor is available, a handle makes a good substitute (Simple Fitness Solutions, n.d.).

Thermoplastic Rubber

This material is often used because it is a cheaper option. Thermoplastic rubber (TPR) is a man-made product with characteristics of both rubber and plastic, which makes it fairly strong. The manufacturing process is cheaper than the extraction of natural rubber, so it is used quite extensively.

It can be recycled, unlike natural rubber, because its block-like structure allows for recrystallization many times over (*What is Thermoplastic Rubber? (TPR)*, 2017).

Extruded Rubber

Extruded or natural rubber comes from rubber trees. The product is described as extruded because it is not molded into its final form like TPR. The soft and pliable rubber compound is fed into a die through an extruder, increasing pressure and temperature along the way to force the rubber through the openings in the die. The finished product is soft and has to be hardened in a process called vulcanization before it can be used (Timco Rubber, n.d.).

The main difference with TPR is in the distance a natural rubber band can stretch before it breaks. TPR can only stretch four or five times its length, while extruded rubber can be stretched up to six times its length. Natural rubber is also less susceptible to light degradation from UV rays (Garage Gym Reviews, n.d.).

Latex

Natural latex comes from the rubber tree in the form of a thick milky liquid. It is harvested by cutting strips of bark from the tree and allowing the liquid to drip into a container placed below the tree.

The harvest is then sent to a processing plant where it undergoes various processes to remove the water and stabilize the product. The concentrated latex contains about 60 percent rubber. Raw materials are then added to it to achieve the desired characteristics for the product.

Natural latex molds itself completely around anything such as plastic tubing dipped into it. Resistance tubes are formed by this process. (Sheppard, 2014). Dipped latex tubing can be stretched up to nine times their length (Garage Gym Reviews, n.d.).

If you have a latex allergy there are fabric alternatives available. The fabric makes the bands a little less stretchy than rubber or latex bands, which makes them ideal for lower body workouts.

Mini Hip Circle Resistance Bands

These sturdy exercise buddies are designed to strengthen the lower body. They are used around the legs, just above the knees, while different movements are performed. They are especially helpful to strengthen the hips and glutes.

A simple example of an exercise where a mini hip circle band is used to great effect is to place the band around your legs just above the knees and place your feet far enough apart so that some tension is detectable in the band. Then start walking forward and feel the tightness in the muscles put to work (Gunsmith Fitness, n.d.). This type of exercise holds great advantages for an older person seeking to regain strength, mobility, and flexibility in the hips. It prevents injuries and also improves balance.

Mini hip circle bands can be purchased in either fabric or non-fabric versions.

RENRANRING Resistance Bands

RENRANRING is a brand that offers latex as well as non-latex options, making their therapy bands a good option for hospitals and other facilities with a no-latex policy.

Online marketplaces like Amazon (Amazon, 2020) and Desertcart (Desertcart, n.d.) offer a whole variety of their products. There are complete sets of tubes with a door anchor, detachable handles, ankle straps, and a carry bag. They also manufacture sets of three open-ended flat bands with or without latex.

Figure 8 Resistance Bands

Also called a figure 8 expander, it is a loop that is fastened together in the middle in a figure eight form with handles on each end. It can be used around the feet or ankles for lower body exercises, around the hands or arms for the upper body, or in a combination of one side around the foot and the other around an arm or in the hand.

They are typically shorter than loop bands and prevent the wear and tear that looping a straight band can cause. The handles make them easier on the hands and also protect the bands from the shoes when looped around a foot.

The construction makes it somewhat easier for a band to snap or pull out of the center fastener, so exercise one arm at a time instead of both simultaneously (Mulrooney, 2011).

Letsfit Resistance Power Loop Bands

Letsfit is a company that specializes in making fitness and health information and accessories available to anyone. They offer sets with power loop bands as well as tubing in all the different strengths. There is also a product specifically developed to prevent rolling up with use (Letsfit, n.d.).

Therapy Bands

Used extensively for physiotherapy and to assist with home rehabilitation after an injury, therapy bands offer mostly light resistance although they are available in different strengths. They are flat bands that are not looped, and the average length is four feet.

They have exceptional elasticity and can be stretched up to 300 percent their own length (Dearden, 2017). Therapy bands are good starting points for resistance training where there is an existing injury, a medical condition, or if the person is frail. They can, however, be difficult to hold on to because they have no handles and no capacity to attach handles (Simple Fitness Solutions, n.d.).

Theraband Resistance Therapy Bands

One of the well-known brands in this field is the company Theraband. They have been around for the last 40 years and pioneered the flat open-ended resistance band as we know it today (Theraband, n.d.). They include tubing in their range. Tubing is the only product that contains latex, while all bands are latex-free (Theraband, n.d.). They also offer a limited range of accessories, such as a wall anchor station for loop bands.

Whatafit Resistance Therapy Bands

The Chinese company Whatafit lists some of its bestseller products as their complete sets of resistance bands (Whatafit, n.d.). Some sets include accessories such as a door anchor, ankle straps, and detachable handles for tubing. They also offer sets of long pull-up bands.

Perfect Peach Resistance Therapy Bands

An online company that took the needs of women specifically to heart, is Perfect Peach Athletics. Their resistance bands sport peach, pink, and lilac color codes instead of the usual colors to denote the different strengths. They also pride themselves on products that are designed to be soft on a woman's skin while not compromising on durability (Perfect Peach Athletics, n.d.). The bands are also offered in a fabric version.

Tribe Resistance Bands

Tribe latex resistance bands are offered in sets as well as single tubes and bands with the usual accessories like a door anchor, detachable handles, and ankle straps (Tribe Fitness USA, n.d.).

Valeo Resistance Bands

The company Valeofit promises affordable prices for good quality with all their merchandise. Their range of bands in different lengths and tubes with accessories is available on Amazon and also offers other rehabilitation products like squeeze balls (Amazon Valeofit Store, 2020).

EDX Resistance Bands

EDX USA has a fairly extensive range of bands, tubing, and accessories available, which grew out of the personal experience of one of their founders. Everything from flat bands to 8-bands, padded detachable handles, and sets are offered (EDX USA, n.d.).

Lux Fitness Resistance Bands

The company Lux Fitness offers wide, elastic bands with non-slip inner layers. The non-slip elastic fabric makes them stronger than plastic or latex and minimizes the possibility of bad smells and skin irritation. Although the bands are marketed as hip, they can be utilized on other parts of the body, according to their website (Lux Fitness, n.d.). Their range also includes tubing and detachable handles.

Ziftex Resistance Bands

This company currently has a limited range of products, which includes a set of looped resistance bands (Ziftex, n.d.).

Physioworks Resistance Bands

Physioworks is an Australian company specializing in a wide range of physiotherapy products. They also have a line of exercise equipment, which includes power loop bands, figure 8 bands, loop bands, and stretch resistance bands as well as accessories like door anchors and detachable handles (Physioworks, n.d.).

8-Shape Resistance Bands

These bands, also called expanders, in the shape of a figure eight, provide a somewhat more challenging workout with some exercises. It is also sometimes known as an ultra toner. They can replace an ordinary looped band that is just twisted into a figure eight, making it easier to keep the shape firmly in place during the exercise because the form is fixed.

Let's look at a couple of easy exercises (Freytag, 2014):

- Put the band in the middle of your shoes with a loop on each foot. Sidestep three or four times to the right and back, then to the left and back. This engages the muscles in the thighs, buttocks, and hips.
- Wear the band in the same way as in the previous exercise, but squat down as low as you can while keeping resistance between your feet tight. Do five to eight repetitions.
- A variation on the exercise above is to stand with your heels together and your toes pointing outwards, before squatting.
- Hold the band in your hands, and pull the loops away from each other across your chest. Keep your back straight, and your shoulders relaxed and down.
- Engage your core muscles in the exercise above by lifting one foot off the ground while pulling the band open.
- Loop one ring around one foot and hold the other ring in your opposite hand. Push your foot away from you while pulling on the band with your arm. Keep your back straight, your shoulders relaxed, and your chin level.

Let your imagination invent more exercises for this versatile resistance band. Many everyday activities can be mimicked while wearing it. If you are traveling and have to keep your luggage as light as possible, an 8-shape band can replace some of the other bands and accessories.

BFR Bands

Simply put, blood flow restriction (BFR) training partially restricts blood flow to certain muscles during exercise to provoke muscle adaptation (BfR Professional, 2018). When used correctly, the restriction band should only obstruct the surface veins without affecting the deeper arteries at all.

According to BfR Professional (2018), the main advantage of this type of training is that the same results can be achieved with lighter workouts as with much heavier routines and weight lifting. They emphasize the need for proper warm-ups before starting occlusion training and to listen to your body and not overdo it because longer sets with shorter rest periods can be performed.

Superpump BFR bands

One of the brands available online through Amazon is Superpump (*Amazon.com : SUPERPUMP BFR BANDS | Simple + Effective Quick-Release Straps for Blood Flow Restriction Training and Kaatsu Style Workouts |*

Arms : Sports & Outdoors, 2020). They offer comfort with a military-grade hook and loop closure for durability.

Resistance Band Rollers

A variation on traditional resistance tubes is adding a roller at each end with a pad on which to kneel or stand in the middle. This allows for a greater variety of exercises.

Foam Rollers

Foam rolling is another technique often used to release tension and increase range of motion. Used as a rehabilitation tool, it has also been added at the end of workouts as part of the cool-down (Victoria, 2016). The roller can be applied to all the points that trigger pain and the amount of pressure is determined by yourself.

According to Anna Victoria (2016), foam rolling or self-myofascial release can be especially beneficial for the lower body, abs, and back, and not much more than a five-minute routine is needed. It helps to increase blood flow and speeds up circulation, thereby preventing and breaking down scar tissue at the sites of injuries.

After a long day, rolling for a few minutes just before going to bed can ease built-up tension and pave the way for a restful night's sleep.

Many different brands are available online and in fitness stores, but if you can't purchase one, there are cheap and easy alternatives (*No Foam Roller? No Problem! Try These Alternatives! | ISSA*, n.d.).

- According to ISSA (n.d.), any ball like a tennis ball can be used as a substitute for a roller. If a tennis ball is too soft, a baseball will also do. The smaller surface of a ball works better when you lie down on the floor or press the ball against a wall. There are also dedicated massage balls available in different shapes, styles, and sizes.
- A kitchen rolling pin with something soft like dishcloths wrapped around it to soften the touch somewhat can also be used.
- A broomstick can target smaller areas and pinpoint scar tissue.
- Any hard bottle or a softer one filled with water will provide the same relief from tension and muscle aches. The harder the object is used, the more intense the pressure will be, and the deeper the massage will be.

Pull-Up Bands

Pull-up bands are the real heavyweights of the resistance band tribe. They have to be long but strong enough to hold an average person's weight and assist with pulling yourself up from the floor for certain exercises.

Grebest is one of the brands available online through Amazon (Amazon, n.d.). They offer lifetime durability in natural latex, with a return policy in case you are not satisfied with the product. The bands are also available in different resistance levels.

Long Bands

Some exercises like squats, pull-ups, and any movement requiring assistance will need a longer band to perform them comfortably. The shorter bands are also not suitable to anchor on a door, for instance.

If you are new to fitness or require a fair amount of assistance, a blue band offering a resistance of around 10 to 15 pounds. That provides a helping hand while still remaining challenging (Set for set, 2019).

They are also sometimes called assistance bands.

Kinetic Leg Resistance Straps

Sometimes foot injuries or certain foot conditions need the foot to remain upright and flat while stretching the Achilles tendon or calf muscle for the exercise to work properly without causing more damage. A resistance band with a strap that goes around the foot at one end is an effective way to ensure this.

It can also be worn while sleeping to keep on providing a gentle stretch to relieve pain caused by stress fractures in the heel and assist with correcting gait problems. It can be very useful when ankle flexibility is an issue (SoCal Health, n.d.).

Door Anchors

For some exercises to be effective, the bands need to be anchored around or under something. If you do not want to go to the trouble of fixing a permanent hook to a wall, there are cheap and easy ways to get around the problem.

A heavy piece of furniture can help you out, but you have to be sure it is really heavy. You do not want a piece of furniture to come flying at you.

A practical way to anchor your bands is by using a door anchor. It consists of a band with a loop at one end, into which a block is put. The band slides under the door with the block at the back of the door, catching there and making it possible to do exercises with heavy tension safely.

The band can also be inserted between the door and the jamb, with the anchor behind the door. This allows for variety in heights (Matt, n.d.).

In a pinch, you could fashion your own anchor out of an old T-shirt or belt just make sure the material is strong enough and that your knots will hold.

Ankle Straps

One of the useful accessories available for resistance bands is a sturdy wide ankle band with a clip attached. It is a safe and comfortable way to do leg exercises, minimizing strain on the ankles.

Handles

Handles are usually found on tubes rather than flat loop bands, although loop bands are occasionally fitted with handles too. The types of exercises usually done with loop bands make handles somewhat awkward to use though. Tubes are also rated for heavier resistance than bands, so handles make it easier to use the tube properly without discomfort (Harwood, 2018).

Handles can be made from hard plastic, or come in padded versions. Padding makes them softer on the hands. Padded handles consist of a nylon webbing pouch with a plastic handle with foam padding around it inside.

If the handle is equipped with a hook to attach it to different tubes, the hooks are manufactured from steel.

Chapter 6:

Resistance Band Series Exercises

I bet you're itching to start applying everything you've learned by now, and you should have all the proper gear in place to do so. It's time to start moving!

Before getting into designing your own workouts or even following along with guided ones, we should pay some attention to all the different movements and their functions. One of the first concepts we need to look at is the different body parts that need to be trained and are grouped together for practical purposes.

The Main Body Parts

We can group exercises for the upper body, core, lower body, back, and abdomen.

Upper Body

The primary body parts and muscles in the upper body include the neck, shoulders, arms, chest, and upper back (Weight Loss Resources UK, n.d.).

Neck

We often don't give our necks a second thought until pain is present, but it is a vital part of our bodies. Weak neck muscles have an important impact on well-being in seniors.

The neck is a conduit between the brain and the spinal cord and there is not much padding in the form of muscles to protect this important passage. Fatigued and weak neck muscles can affect nerve impulses and hamper functioning and movement. Compromised neck muscles can even affect the quality of breathing (Kelso, n.d.).

Exercising and stretching the neck muscles are super easy and quick, and you reap immediate benefits in feeling better.

- Chin on chest: Bend your head forwards and try to push your chin into your chest. Hold for a couple of seconds and relax. For added oomph, fasten one end of your resistance band around your forehead and hook the other end around an anchor before pulling forward against it.

- Look up towards the ceiling, tilting your head back as far as is comfortable for you to do. With the resistance band positioned as in the previous exercise, you can also pull against the band to make the exercise a bit more challenging.
- Move your head from one shoulder to the other, flexing your neck as far as possible without pain. Pull against the resistance band if it doesn't hurt you to do so.
- Look to the right and the left as if you are about to cross a busy street. Turn your head as far as possible to each side and use your resistance band here (Kelso, n.d.).

Shoulders

The main muscles in the shoulders are the deltoids, which are at the top, and the rotator cuffs at the bottom (Weight Loss Resources UK, n.d.).

As we age, we often lose strength and toning in the upper body quickly because we don't lift and push things as often anymore while our legs still carry our body weight for a workout.

- Shoulder press for the deltoids: Use a long band or tube and stand in the center of it. Raise your hands to shoulder height. With the band behind your arms, bend your elbows at 90 degrees with palms facing outwards. Straighten your arms

towards the ceiling. If it is impossible to get your arms into a straight position, you can lighten the resistance (Dick's Pro Tips, 2019).
- External rotation for the rotator cuff: Attach your resistance band to an anchor at belly button height. Stand perpendicular to the band and take it in your outside hand. Pull the band away from the anchor while keeping your elbow against your body. You can pinch a towel between your body and elbow to make sure your elbow doesn't move away (Set for Set, 2017).
- Wall crawl: Attach a short looped band around your wrists and lean your forearms against a wall. Keeping your shoulder blades as low as possible, crawl your forearms up the wall until the band is at eye level (Set for Set, 2017).
- Shrug: Stand with your arms by your sides. Pull your shoulders up as high as possible, squeezing your shoulder blades together at the top. For added resistance, you can fasten two bands to something near the floor and hold them taut before pulling your shoulders up.
- Front raise: Kneel with a resistance band looped under one knee. Pull the band straight up to shoulder height with one hand. Lower the arm slowly and repeat with the other arm (8fit Team, n.d.).

- Lateral raise: Do exactly the same as in the previous exercise, but pull the band out to the side, perpendicular to the body (8fit Team, n.d.).
- Seated row: Sit on the floor with your legs straight out in front of you. Loop the band around your feet and pull your hands back to your sides (8fit Team, n.d.).
- Lawnmower: This exercise imitates starting a lawnmower and is extremely easy to perform with resistance bands. Anchor the band in front of you or stand on it. Keep it fairly short and pull backward and up, as if trying to start a lawnmower with a pull cord. Alternate sides. It is also good for the back (Picincu, 2020).

Arms

An arm workout also benefits the shoulders, chest, and back. Only one band is needed for all the exercises.

Try to do ten repetitions. The seventh and eighth should feel challenging, but you should still be able to finish the set. If you glide through all of the repetitions without feeling tired, it is time to move up to a band with more resistance (Eisinger, 2019).

- Seated biceps curl: Sit on a chair with one end of the band under your left foot. Take the other end in your right hand and rest your right elbow on your thigh. The band should be taut. Keep your back straight and pull your right hand up towards your right shoulder with the palm facing upwards. The bicep muscle is located on the front of the upper arm, and you should feel it working to pull the band up (Eisinger, 2019).
- Reverse curl: Do exactly the same as in the previous exercise, but turn your palm to face down (Eisinger, 2019).

- Flexion: Sit down and anchor the resistance band in front of you, level with your knees. Place your hands on your knees, hold one end of the band in each hand with your palms facing upwards. Flex your wrists upward, pulling the band and feeling the muscles in both the wrist and the forearm contracting (Eisinger, 2019).
- Archery pull: This exercise imitates pulling a bow to shoot an arrow and reaches muscles that are not used in many everyday activities. Hold a looped band out in front of you perpendicular to your body. Pull the front end away from you as if drawing a bowstring. Hold the position for a few seconds and relax (Barber, 2018).
- Tricep extension: The triceps are at the back of the arms. Stand with one foot slightly in front of the other and with the center of the band under the back foot. Hold the ends of the bands in your hands and pull them up straight above your head. Slowly lower the ends behind your head until your elbows are bent 90 degrees. Move your arms up again slowly (Eisinger, 2019).
- Chair triceps dip: Anchor a band at a point high against a door or wall. Sit on a chair in front of the band and take the ends of the band in your hands. Gently pull down as far as possible (Eisinger, 2019).

- Overhead triceps extension: Stand on the center of the resistance band and pull the ends up until your hands are over your shoulders with your elbows pointing forward. Extend your arms in a straight line and bring them down again. Repeat five to eight times (Biswas, 2018).

Chest

The main muscles in the chest are the pectorals. They connect the front of the chest with the bones in your shoulder and upper arm.

- Chest press: Wrap a band around your body, chest height. Push the band out in front of you until your arms are straight. Hold for a few seconds and relax (Rubberbanditz, 2019).
- Incline press: Do exactly the same as in the previous exercise, but push your arms up at an angle instead of straight out in front of you (Rubberbanditz, 2019).
- Chest fly: Loop a resistance band around your body and stretch your arms out in front of you. Keeping tension tight in the band, pull your arms back as far as possible. Hold for a few seconds and relax (Rubberbanditz, 2019).
- Reverse chest fly: Do the same exercise as above, but start with your arms at the back and bring them forward slowly (Rubberbanditz, 2019).

- Pull down: Anchor the band high enough so that it is pulled taut when you kneel holding the ends above your head. Bring your arms down to shoulder height, hold the position for a few seconds, and gently let your arms go up again (*Resistance Band Lat Pulldown*, n.d.).

Lower Body

The lower body includes the knees, which are a problem for many older people, as well as the pelvis. Weak pelvic floor muscles can cause bladder and bowel problems for women especially and are often neglected in exercise routines.

While the knees have tendons and not muscles, weak knees affect the strength of the legs and hips (Young, 2020). Women are quite susceptible to knee problems in later years, because of their wider hips. Wearing high heels in youth can come back to haunt you later because this constant elevated foot position tends to shift weight to the knees.

- The gas pedal exercise: This exercise was discussed in Chapter Three as part of the warm-up routine.
- Leg press: This exercise is best done in a seated position to keep the upper body and torso still and make balancing easy. Wrap the band around your feet and hold the ends just above thigh height. Push your legs straight out in front of you and bring them back again to the starting position. The exercise can also be done laying down if preferred (Nunez, 2018).
- Squats: Loop a resistance band around your shins and stand with your feet wide enough that some resistance from the band can be felt. Keeping your back straight, squat down with hips extended to the back while holding the distance between your feet. Hold your arms out in front of you or clasp your hands for balance. Come back up slowly in a controlled movement. When your thigh muscles are strong

enough, you can widen the distance between your feet to do a sumo squat (Nunez, 2018).
- Squat shuffle: Place the resistance band just above your knees. Slowly go down into a squat stance, pushing your hips out and bending your knees. Keep your back straight, your feet flat, and your toes in line with your hips. Shuffle to one side and back (Nunez, 2018).
- Forward lunge: Lunges are an old favorite in workouts because they engage almost the entire lower body, as well as the core. Loop a band under one foot and grasp each end in a hand. Take a big step forward with one foot until the other knee almost touches the ground. Keep tension in the band all the time. Push yourself back up again to the starting position (Rubberbanditz, 2019).
- Sidestep: Loop a resistance band around your ankles while your feet are shoulder-width apart. Take a large step to one side, well outside your shoulders. Pause there for a moment, then step with the other foot in the same direction. Keep stepping for three or four paces before returning to the starting point (Rubberbanditz, 2019).
- Leg curls: This exercise concentrates on the hamstrings. Sit on a chair and anchor your band in front of you. Loop the other end around one

ankle. Keep your feet together and pull your legs back as far as they can go before returning to the starting position (Nunez, 2018).
- Leg abduction: Lie on your back with a band looped around your feet and the ends in your hands. Keep your elbows on the ground beside you. Open your legs wider than your hips and bring your feet back again to the starting position (Spark People, n.d.).
- Hip extension: Loop the band around your ankles. Extend one leg behind you as far as possible, keeping it straight. Return to the starting position slowly and in a controlled manner (Nunez, 2018).

The Core

Effective core training strengthens much more than just your six-pack or rectus abdominis. It engages all the muscles that wrap around the abdominal area, as well as the pelvis, hips, back, and glutes (Atemi Sports, 2019).

- Chair sit-up: Sit on a chair with a band looped around your ankles. Keep your lower back as straight as possible, and bend forward to move your chest towards your thighs. Keep your feet flat on the ground and keep the tension in the band constant. Come back up slowly and repeat five to eight times (Atemi Sports, 2019).

- Reverse wood chop: Anchor the band and hold the other end with both hands. Bend your knees slightly and pull the band across your body and up. Return to the starting position, keeping full control of the movement (Train With Me Fitness Inc, n.d.).
- Side bend: Grasp the band at the ends and extend your arms above your head while keeping the band stretched tight. Bend to one side and keep the tension in the band. Keep the position for a few seconds before bending to the other side. Keep your body straight all the time (Fit Carrots, n.d.).
- Pelvic lift: This exercise is performed while lying on the back with a resistance band looped around the knees. Lift your hips into a bridge position and gently push your knees out against the resistance of the band. Repeat the movement with toes pointing inward and outward (Watkins, 2014).
- Push-ups: Loop a resistance band around your upper body, under your arms. Lie down on your stomach and push your upper body up on your arms. You can also bend your knees instead of keeping your legs straight to make the exercise somewhat easier (Fit Carrots, n.d.).

The Back

Many back pain sufferers will find relief when their back muscles and other supporting muscles are strengthened enough to carry their weight with ease. Resistance band training is an excellent and safe way to achieve this.

- Lat pull-down: Loop a resistance band around your wrists and extend your arms above your head. Push your hands away from each other while lowering the band behind your shoulders. Return to the starting position (Cordeau, n.d.).
- Pull-apart: Hold the ends of a resistance band with your arms stretched out in front of you, and the band pulled tight. Pull your hands away from each other while keeping your back absolutely straight. Return to the starting position (Cordeau, n.d.).
- Back fly lying: Stand with both feet on a band and tilt your body forwards. Extend your arms in front of your knees with palms facing each other. Pull your arms backward and out behind your body as far as possible. Keep the position for a few seconds before returning to the starting position (Patricie K, n.d.).
- Bent over rows: Place your feet on the band, hip-width apart. Bend forward at the waist and grasp the handles. Pull them up in a rowing motion with palms facing the body. Keep the back straight and lift the elbows towards the ceiling (Spark People, n.d.).

- Deadlift: Stand on the band and hold the ends with your palms facing backward. Push your hips down until you feel your hamstrings stretch. Keep your torso and back straight while pushing upright again slowly (Rubberbanditz, 2019).

The Abdominal Area

Muscles in the abdominal area influence breathing, posture, stability, and balance. When they are strong, everyday activities like bending down to tie your shoe or swinging a golf club become much easier.

Strong abdominal muscles can alleviate lower back pain and assist in maintaining the correct weight (EFM Healthclubs, 2018).

- Standing knee raising: Stand with your feet slightly wider than shoulder-width and place a resistance band around the middle of your feet. Lift one leg to your chest and try to touch your knee to your elbow without rounding your shoulders. Alternate legs (Mateo, 2017).
- Banana rolls: The trick with this exercise is never to let your hands and feet touch the floor. Lie on your front with hands and feet lifted off the floor. Position a resistance band around your ankles. Roll over onto your back, keeping

the tension in the band. Roll back to your stomach while still keeping hands and feet clear of the floor (Mateo, 2017).

- Bicycle crunches: Loop a resistance band around the middle of your feet. Sit on the floor with bent knees and heels touching the floor. Lean back until you can feel your abdominal muscles working. Hook your fingertips behind your ears and twist your body to touch your right elbow to your left knee while straightening your right leg. Do the same with the other arm and leg to complete one repetition. Repeat five to eight times (Mateo, 2017).
- Side plank: This exercise could be fairly difficult for beginners, and you should listen to your body when attempting it. Pain anywhere means your muscles are not ready yet. Lie down on your side with one foot stacked on top of the other and a resistance band around your ankles. Push yourself up on the bottom arm with the heel of the bottom foot touching the floor. Lift the top leg up stretching the band, and try to hold the position for 30 seconds before relaxing and doing the same on the other side (Mateo, 2017).
- Plank hold: Another variation on the plank exercise is to loop a resistance band around your waist. Kneel on the floor with your palms

down, and thumbs hooked into the band. Support your body on one knee and push the opposite leg out straight to the back. Straighten the other leg as well and hold the position for a few seconds (Biswas, 2018).
- Spiderman push-up: This is another exercise that can be quite difficult in the beginning. Start in a push-up position with a resistance band around the middle of your feet. As you go down towards the floor, pull your right knee up towards your elbow. Alternate legs (Mateo, 2017).
- Sit-ups: Anchor the resistance band in front of you and lie down on the floor with the ends of the band in your hands. Bend your knees slightly and keep your feet flat on the floor. Pull yourself upright into a sitting position with the aid of the band and keep your back straight and your shoulders relaxed and down (Mateo, 2017).

Golfing Exercises

Although a golf club is not part of the body, ardent golfers in their senior years with enough leisure time to pursue this pastime might argue.

Resistance band training is especially beneficial to golfers to create consistency in their game or make more powerful swings. Even professional golfers have discovered the benefits of resistance bands in recent years, and trainers never leave home without them (Herman, 2017).

Targeted Warm-Ups

With resistance bands, you can target and tailor your warm-up routine to focus on any body part or muscle that is nursing an injury or is not as strong as you would like it to be.

The buzz word is prehabilitation, which is a shortened form of preventative rehabilitation. Exercises in this category not only warm up the targeted muscles and joints but also strengthen them at the same time to prevent injury further down the line. Shoulder rotator cuffs are an excellent example of the type of body part where golfers can use prehab to great advantage (Herman, 2017).

If you have to start a game while still sore from the previous day's activities, resistance band warm-ups at light resistance will help you ease into movement gradually and prevent injury.

Joint Stability

Stability and flexibility go hand in hand and become more and more important in later years. Golfers undergo a particular type of wear and tear to their joints due to repetitive movements, and loop bands can isolate the small groups of muscle around joints, to stabilize them (Herman, 2017).

The elasticity of the bands also supports a full range of motion to increase and maintain mobility in ways that weights and other types of exercises just cannot do.

The All-Important Swing

What is a golfer without his swing, you might ask? Whether you just want to improve or if there is an issue with your technique, resistance bands are perfectly suited to mold motor patterns and movements.

Trainers often use a type of reverse technique when a specific technical issue has to be modified. If the negative movement is initiated with a resistance band, the golfer is forced to move in the opposite direction, thereby executing the correct movement. Through cell memory, the new and correct motor pattern is laid down in the brain, and a revised technique starts taking shape (Herman, 2017).

Being so portable and lightweight, the bands can be carried into any change room and used on-demand without assistance from anyone else.

Fitness

As with any sport, golf requires a manner of fitness that is suitable for the demands of the sport. There are distances to be walked between holes to get the full benefit of being outside in the fresh air. If you do not have the luxury of a caddy, the heavy golf bag must also be carried around.

Arms and shoulders getting tired halfway through the game might just cost you the bottle of vintage wine up for grabs as a prize for the winner.

Let's look at some exercises that are recommended for golfers.

- Golfer's wood chop: Anchor your band behind you at about the point from where you would swing your golf club to play. Take the other end in both hands and perform a diagonal downward movement as if you are swinging a club. Make sure you stand far enough from the anchor point to create a fair amount of resistance against the downward swing and try

to do it faster every time for two repetitions before switching sides. Perform three sets. Focus on controlled movement, not the type of strength that will hit the ball into the next county (Bowden, 2015)
- To strengthen the 'pushing' part of your golf swing, do the same exercise as above but only use your trailing arm (Bowden, 2015).
- The 'pulling' part of the swing can be exercised by repeating the previous exercise, but this time using your lead arm (Bowden, 2015).
- To work on your follow-through, anchor the band low and take the other end with your swing hand. Extend your arm upwards in the follow-through movement while pulling against the resistance of the band (Bowden, 2015).
- The impact with which the ball is struck can be exercised by taking hold of the band with the back arm and pulling it forward and downward, extending the triceps to the impact position (Bowden, 2015).

If you do these golf-specific exercises before going onto the green, you will have a great warm-up and be ready to play the game at your best.

Adding Accessories

You can add accessories like balls and dumbbells to many of the exercises described above to create variety and possibly even make them effective in a shorter time, depending on your own strength and where you are in your fitness journey.

Balls

Fitness or balance balls are a good accessory to your workout to help with stability and core strength. Balance ball resistance kits are available that consist of two resistance bands that fit over the ball for a more challenging workout.

- Reclining fly exercise: Sit on the ball and hold on to the ends of the resistance band. Roll back until your back is on the ball and keep your feet flat on the ground. Straighten your arms, pulling

on the bands. Hold the top position for a few seconds and relax (Skimble, n.d.).
- Upright fly: Do the same exercise as above, but stay upright. This version might be easier for anyone with back problems (Skimble, n.d.).
- Chest press: Sit down on the ball with the ends of the bands in your hands. Pull the bands up and over your chest. Lower your arms, but no lower than shoulder height (Waehner, 2019).
- Bench press: Do the same exercise as above while lying down on the ball (Waehner, 2019.

Dumbbells

Widely used in strength training, these weights come in different sizes and can be used for a variety of different exercises. They consist of a handle with a weight on each side. The weights can be fixed or removable.
- Chest press: Loop a band around your back. Take the dumbbells one in each hand and press the band out with your hands on the inside of the band. Push the band and dumbbells up above your head and hold for a few seconds before relaxing (Skimble, n.d.).
- Chest fly: Lie on your back and loop a band around your wrists. Hold the dumbbells in your hands and rest your arms straight out to your sides at shoulder height. The band should be

taut. Lift both arms straight up and bring them back down slowly (Skimble, n.d.).
- Lateral raises: Stand on the band and take a dumbbell and an end of the band in each hand. Raise your arms to the sides, up to shoulder height, and hold for a few seconds before relaxing (Bentley, 2016).
- Frontal raise: Do exactly the same exercise as above, but raise your arms in front of you instead of to the sides.
- Biceps curl: Stand in the middle of a band with a dumbbell in each hand and loop the ends of the band over the dumbbells. Pull the dumbbells up to shoulder height and hold for a few seconds before releasing (Brathwaite, 2018).

Chapter 7:

Sample Core Workouts

In this chapter, you will find examples of core workouts that will help you achieve your desired results. It will help you see the pattern of a successful core workout and empower you to design your routines.

Remember, it is your life, make it interesting! Enjoy the road to greater health, fitness, and happiness. These examples are just starting points. Take a look at all the exercises in the book and play around with them until you have the perfect combination for you.

Core Workout 1

There are three exercises in this workout: The bicycle crunch, the mountain climber, and the hip thrust. Do them one after the other. Use 45 seconds per exercise with 15 seconds of rest in between. That brings you to a total workout time of nine minutes.

Bicycle Crunch

This vigorous exercise was discussed in Chapter Six under workouts for the abdominal area, but let's recap quickly.

It is best done sitting on the floor with bent knees and heels touching the floor. Position the resistance band around the middle of your feet and lean back until you can feel your abdominal muscles tugging and stretching. Keep them tight.

Hook your fingertips loosely behind your ears and twist your body to touch your right elbow to your left knee while straightening your right leg. Do the same with the other arm and leg to complete one repetition (Mateo, 2017).

Adapt your tempo to your fitness level and any physical constraints you might have. If you feel up for it, you can increase the intensity by holding a weight like a dumbbell or even just a can of tinned food in your hands while touching your elbows to your knees.

Mountain Climber

The traditional mountain climber exercise is performed quickly. Adding the resistance of a band makes it slower and far more intense and effective. It also adds benefits for the hips.

Get down on the floor in a push-up position, with a mini band around your ankles. Pull one knee up towards your chest as if you are climbing a rock. Return to the starting position and repeat with the other leg to complete one repetition (Gomez, 2017).

Hip Thrust

Hip thrusts specifically target all the gluteus muscles in particular. The exercise isolates them in a more effective way than more general hip movements can.

Lie on your back with the band looped over your thighs. Pin the ends of the band on the sides of your body with your hands. Keep your knees bent and your feet flat on the floor. Push your hips up against the band.

If you want to add weight, you can put a dumbbell under the band on your tummy (Fit Carrots, n.d.).

Core Workout 2

This workout has four exercises: The low-high chop, the side plank row, the high leg raise, and the high plank row. They are to be performed as supersets consisting of three sets each with 12 to 15 repetitions in each set. By the seventh repetition of each movement, it should start feeling challenging; otherwise, you will have to increase the repetitions.

The total workout time should be 10 to 15 minutes.

Low-High Chop

The wood chop was discussed in the previous chapter under core exercises. It can be done from either a high or low starting point. For the greatest effectiveness in core training, it is best to start it from below.

Anchor the band close to the floor. Bend down and take hold of the other end with both hands. With slightly bent knees, pull the band across your body and up as if you are raising an ax to chop wood. Return to the low starting position, keeping full control of the movement (Train With Me Fitness Inc, n.d.). Controlled movement and a full range of motion are very important in this exercise.

To add intensity, you can hold a dumbbell in your hands and lift that as well.

Side Plank Row

Lie down on the floor on your side and in the plank position. The band must be attached to a point close to the floor level. Hold the ends of the band in your top hand and raise yourself into a plank. Perform a rowing motion with the top arm (Men's Health, 2011).

High Leg Raise

Lie on your back with a mini band looped around your ankles and your heels on the floor. Lift one leg as high as possible against the band's resistance while keeping the other leg still and your shoulders firmly on the floor.

Do the same with the other leg to complete one repetition (Atemi Sports, 2019).

High Plank Row

The trusty plank exercise for core strength works on more than 20 muscles at the same time. It minimizes the chances for a back injury and does not hold the risks of hip stress, unlike sit-ups (Andersen, 2014).

It is advisable to master the basic plank before attempting to add the row.

Anchor a band low on the floor in front of you and get into plank position while holding the ends of the band. Bend your elbow and pull your arm slowly towards the ceiling, all the while working against the resistance of the band. The elbow should remain close to your side. Repeat with the other side to complete one repetition.

Use a dumbbell in the hand that is lifting to add intensity (Andersen, 2014).

Core Workout 3

As with the previous sample workout, the four exercises in this example should be performed as supersets consisting of three sets each, with 12 to 15 repetitions in each set. By the seventh repetition of each movement, it should start feeling challenging; otherwise, you will have to increase the repetitions.

The exercises are the bicycle crunch, the mountain climber, the torso rotation, and the side plank reach.

Bicycle Crunch

This exercise remains the same as explained in the first core sample workout.

Mountain Climber

This exercise also remains the same as explained in the first core sample workout.

Torso Rotation

The same exercise was discussed in chapter three as the twister exercise and done slowly like described there, it is an excellent warm-up movement.

It has its place in any core routine though, because once the muscles are warmed up, the exercise can be performed somewhat faster for a more thorough workout.

The muscles targeted are the abdominals that provide support to the whole abdominal area. Weakness in these muscles can have a significant impact on back health.

The obliques next to the abdominals are conditioned at the same time. They play a stabilizing role and are just as important for posture and overall health (Train With Me Fitness Inc, n.d.).

While the body rotation done with only a resistance band provides a good workout, holding a dumbbell while rotating will add intensity when your fitness level allows it.

The exercise can also be done in a seated position if preferred, and the dumbbell can be substituted for a medicine ball or any other fairly heavy object such as a bag of flour or cans of tinned food.

You should sit with your feet off the ground and rotate from hip to hip (Train With Me Fitness Inc, n.d.).

Side Plank Reach

Start in a side plank position. With your free hand, hold on to a resistance band that's anchored at a low point behind your back. Pull the band under your body while rotating your rib cage at the same time so that you end up looking down at the floor. It is the same motion as if starting a lawnmower.

Keep your core muscles tight the whole time to prevent your body from rotating too far, and have you ending up flat on the floor.

For added intensity, you can hold a dumbbell in the same hand as the rope (Train With Me Fitness Inc, n.d.).

Other Exercises to Mix and Match

Many of the exercises already discussed in earlier chapters can be swapped out for great core workouts.

Mini-band exercises to consider are the banded squat, mountain climber, bicycle crunch, clamshell, glute bridge, hip thrust, lateral walk, leg abduction, psoas march, and push-ups. Let's look at them!

- Clamshell: This is a great exercise not only for strengthening the hip and core muscles but also for easing tension in the lower back. Lie on your side with your legs stacked and your knees bent at a 45-degree angle. Loop a resistance band around your legs above the knees. Rest your head on your lower arm and steady yourself with your upper arm to help stabilize your hips. Pull your belly button in towards your spine. Raise your top leg as high as possible without moving your hips or lifting your shoulders off the floor. Hold for 10 to 15 seconds and return to the starting position.

- Psoas march: The psoas muscle is one of the hip flexors and influences balance and mobility greatly. To do the exercise, you should lie down on your back with your hips up in a vertical position, your knees bent, and your feet flexed so your toes point to the ceiling. Loop a resistance band around your feet. Take a deep breath and while exhaling, stretch one leg out in front of you and lower it to the lowest point where you can still control the movement. The other leg should remain still, as should your ribcage, shoulders, and pelvis. For added intensity, you could lie with your head close enough to a wall to press your palms against the wall behind your head, fingers pointing towards the floor (Callaway, 2018).

For some exercises, the assistance of a pull-up band is required. These are longer and stronger bands, but they make excellent aids when an extra helping hand is needed.

Here are a few to get you started:

- Band-assisted pistol squats: If you're feeling adventurous and strong, you can try this one-legged squat. Experts warn, however, that you have to be sure you have the strength to complete at least three sets of 15 regular squats before even attempting to do a pistol squat (Carpenter, 2020). Anchor your band high up in front of you and take hold of the ends with both hands. Lift one foot and go down in a squat on the other leg while holding on to the band. Keep your core muscles engaged and your back and ankles straight. In the beginning, you can place a low chair behind you and go down to the chair until you're strong enough to do it without any halfway stop.
- Band-assisted pull-ups: Pull-ups test the back and arms and the use of a resistance band can make the exercise considerably easier to perform. Anchor the band in front of you. The length should be such that your feet do not touch the ground if you stand on the band. Hold on to a bar or something similar above your head and pull your body up as far as possible. Ideally, you should be able to elevate your whole head and neck above the bar. Use

smooth movements, no jerks. Don't lift your chin and strain your neck, let your arms, shoulder, and back do the work. Lower yourself slowly again (Arana, 2019).

- Stationary band-resisted sprints: Bands can be used either as assistance or resistance. For this exercise, the resistance will be utilized. It is an excellent way to increase stamina and endurance and will also assist in burning calories if you want to manage your weight. Simply anchor your band behind you and loop the band around your waist. Then try as hard as you can to run forward, straining against the band. For added resistance, you can add a mini-band above your knees as well (Pridgett, 2019).
- Assisted hip hinge: This exercise focuses on the backside of the core muscles. It is also sometimes called the dowel rod hinge. The muscles targeted are essential for everyday activities where hips are bent, such as picking something up from the floor. The bending movement must come from the hips and not the waist. Place a band around your waist and anchor the band behind you. When you pull against the band, it will help you into a bent position. You have to engage your core muscles to come upright again while keeping your back straight. You must feel your hamstrings

contracting during the movement. Do not let your knees go past your toes (The Prehab Guys, n.d.).

- Assisted skater squats: This exercise is not only good for the hips and legs but also promotes ankle stability. It is quite a vigorous movement. Loop a mini-band around above your knees. Then jump lightly from side to side, controlling your landing tightly and landing softly. Keep the tension in the band, and do not close the gap between your knees (Lugo, 2017).

You now have a solid foundation from which you can start a proper workout program, but also begin building and designing your own similar workouts according to your preferences, physical condition, and lifestyle.

Don't hesitate to begin mixing and matching these movements into fun and interesting groupings that will keep you excited when you think about your exercise program.

Chapter 8:

Designing Your Own Programs

Now we have come to the really exciting and fun part of the book! You know enough of resistance training now to start putting together your own routines. This is where you get to mix and match any exercises that work for you.

I have a couple of suggestions to get you started, but you are the one in the driving seat from here on.

Two Workouts per Week Program

Day One

The exercises should be performed as supersets, consisting of three sets with 10 to 15 repetitions each. The workout should take about 40 minutes.

- Chest press: One version of this exercise was explained in chapter six, but there are other ways of doing it just as effectively. It can be done in a standing, sitting, or lying down position. Instead of pushing your arms out, you can move your body. Anchor the band near the floor and grab hold of the ends. Move your body forward into a lunge position and pull the bands with you until your arms are parallel to the floor at shoulder height. This is a forward and upward movement at the same time (Hoffman, 2020).
- Standing row: This exercise provides a thorough workout for the shoulders and upper back. Anchor the band at chest height and hold the ends so that your hands are slightly in from shoulder width. Stretch your arms out and pull the band towards your belly button while allowing your hands to move away from each other. Stop after reaching your body and return to the starting position. Concentrate on keeping your head and neck relaxed and allow your shoulder blades free movement (The Movement Fix, 2018).
- Glute bridge: The trusty and simple glute bridge in its basic form as discussed in an earlier chapter is a very versatile movement that can be performed in a variety of ways (Salyer, 2016).

When the toes are pointed outward instead of facing forward, a different set of the glutes receive the workout. For more variations, the heels can be pressed down and the toes lifted, or the toes can be pressed down and the heels lifted. The movement can also be performed with only one foot on the floor and the other leg stretched straight up. Placing a weight on your abdomen during the exercise immediately ramps up the intensity (Salyer, 2016).

- Lateral walk: Also known as monster walks and banded shuffles, these mini-band side steps can prevent or alleviate knee pain when performed correctly. There are variations on the basic version discussed earlier in the book. If you use a large band rather than a mini-band and stand on it with the loop crossed in front of you, you engage your shoulders as well. You could also combine the walk with weights in the hands and another mini-band looped around the wrists (Maximum Training Solutions, 2016).
- Arnold press: This all-round multi-joint exercise has not cropped up before in our discussions. Stand or sit with a straight back and loop a mini-band around your wrists. You can either hold a weight in each hand or do the movement without additional weights. Start with your hands on your shoulders and lift your arms until

they are straight while rotating your palms. When you get to the top of the movement, your palms should be facing each other. You can also do one arm at a time or alternate them (*Arnold Press - How To Do It*, n.d.).

- Banded squat: This exercise was discussed in Chapter Six.
- Mountain climber: This exercise was discussed in the third core workout in Chapter Seven.
- Side plank row: This exercise was discussed in Chapter Seven and does require some level of fitness before attempting.

Day Two

The exercises should be performed as supersets, consisting of three sets with 10 to 12 repetitions each. The workout should take about 40 minutes.

- Kneeling pull-down: This exercise was discussed in chapter six. It is worth noting that it can be done by either standing on one knee or both.
- Split squat: Place the middle part of one foot on a band and place the other foot a step behind. Pull the band up towards your shoulders with your elbows pointing towards the floor. Bend both knees to go down in a lunge position before coming upright again (Skimble, n.d.).

- Chest press: As done in day one's program.
- Single-leg deadlift: A variation on the explanation in chapter six is to do the deadlift with only one leg. Loop a resistance band around your ankles. Bend one knee slightly and extend the other leg behind you to help keep your balance. Hold for a few seconds and return to the starting position (Soto, 2018).
- Overhead press: This is an excellent way to tone and strengthen shoulders and arms. Stand on a resistance band with your feet shoulder-width apart. Hold the ends of the band and raise your hands to your shoulders and elbows out to the side. Then raise your arms straight up, working against the resistance of the band. Lower your arms again to shoulder height and repeat the exercise (Sworkit Wellness, n.d.).
- Hip thrust: A slight variation on the version that was discussed in the previous chapter is to sit on the floor with your shoulders and upper arms resting on something like a bed or soft chair. Loop a band around your thighs and under your shoes. Thrust your hips upward so that your body pulls into a straight line, except for your knees that remain bent at a 90-degree angle. Keep your back straight, and imagine you squeeze a coin between your buttocks as you lift your hips. You could also kneel with the band

anchored behind you and lean forward before thrusting your hips out, or stand bent at the waist while pulling the band forward between your legs and pushing yourself upright (BIQ Band Training, 2020).
- Bicycle crunch: This is a staple exercise that crops up in many workout routines. See the discussion in the previous chapter.
- High-low chop: Doing the movement this way round is exactly the opposite of the low-high chop that was discussed in the second sample core workout in the previous chapter.

Three Workouts per Week Program

Day One

The exercises should be performed as supersets, consisting of three sets with 10 to 12 repetitions each. Make sure the seventh repetition becomes challenging. The workout should take about 40 minutes.

- Quadruped kickback: The exercise is also known as quadruped hip extension or glute kickback. It is one of the easier movements for beginners or people without much physical strength. Kneel on the floor and place your hands under your shoulders. Keep your knees positioned under your hips. Lift your knee until your upper leg is parallel with the floor while keeping your knee still bent at a 90-degree angle. Then straighten your leg completely before reversing the process (Williams, 2020).

- Single-leg deadlift: The same as in the previous routine.
- Face pull: Contrary to what the name might suggest, this has nothing to do with your expression. It is basically a shoulder and back strengthening exercise which is done by pulling a band towards your face. Looped bands work best. Anchor it at head height and pull your elbows back, keeping them shoulder height. As your hands get closer to your face, you also pull them apart from each other. Then move back to the starting position in a controlled, smooth movement (Rusin, 2017).
- Push-ups: These need no introduction and have been discussed earlier in the book.
- Standing row: See earlier discussion in the section about day one of the previous programs.
- Banded squat: See the discussion on lower body exercises in chapter six.

- Hip raise: This is just another name for the hip thrust exercise that was discussed earlier.
- Bicycle crunch: See earlier discussions.

Day Two

The exercises should be performed as supersets, consisting of three sets with 10 to 12 repetitions each. Make sure the seventh repetition becomes challenging. The workout should take about 40 minutes.

- Skater squats: This exercise was discussed at the end of the previous chapter.
- Pull-through: When doing hip hinges, it is easy to fall into movement patterns that do not have the desired effect. The pull-through exercise that is done with a long band can prevent that. When done regularly, it will reinforce the correct way of movement for healthy and strong hips. Anchor the band behind you. Bend over and pull the band forward between your knees, locking your hands in place around it. Take a couple of steps forward and feel how the band wants to pull you back. Keep your back straight and allow your hips to go up to the maximum flexion point for your flexibility. Then push yourself upright by using your feet, still keeping your back straight (Barbara M, 2019).

- Hip thrust: See this exercise in the first workout program.
- Chest press: See the discussion in the first program, for the routine on day one.
- Arnold press: See earlier discussions.
- Standing wide row: An alternative to the rowing exercise discussed earlier is to stand with one foot a few steps in front of the other. The forward leg should be the opposite of your working arm. Pull the band towards you while rotating your torso and keeping your elbow flared out (*Alternative Exercises Row*, n.d.).
- Torso rotation: See earlier discussions.
- Side plank reach: See earlier discussions.
- Mountain climber: See earlier discussions.

Day Three

The exercises should be performed as a circuit, starting with the first exercise and ending with the last one, before going back to number one. The time for the workout should be about 36 minutes.

- Push-up: See earlier discussions.
- Glute bridge: See earlier discussions.
- Bicycle crunch: See earlier discussions.
- Banded squat: See earlier discussions.
- Lateral walk: See earlier discussions.

- Band pull-apart: Stand or sit up straight with a band looped around your hands. Pull your hands away from each other as far as you can and hold the position for a couple of seconds. Squeeze your shoulder blades together while doing this. You can also try to pull diagonally instead of in a straight line, as well as holding your arms at different heights to change the degree of difficulty (Coachmag, n.d.).
- Overhead press: See earlier discussions.
- Biceps curl: See earlier discussions.
- Bent-over rear delt fly: See earlier discussions.

Four Workouts per Week Program

Day One

The exercises should be performed as supersets, consisting of three sets with 10 to 12 repetitions each. Make sure the seventh repetition becomes challenging. The workout should take about 40 minutes.

- Band-assisted pull-up: See earlier discussions.
- Push-up: See earlier discussions.
- Arnold press: See earlier discussions.
- Face pull: See earlier discussions.

- High curl: Anchor the band in front of you at eye level. Hold the ends and step back until you can feel the tension in the band. Pull the band towards you, bending your elbows at a 90-degree angle and keeping your back straight and your core muscles tight (Rubberbanditz, 2019)
- Overhead extension: See earlier discussions.
- High-low chop: See earlier discussions.
- Mountain climber: See earlier discussions.

Day Two

The exercises should be performed as supersets, consisting of three sets with 10 to 12 repetitions each. Make sure the seventh repetition becomes challenging. The workout should take about 40 minutes.

- Single-leg bench squat: See earlier discussions.
- Split squat: See earlier discussions.
- Banded squat: See earlier discussions.
- Mountain climber: See earlier discussions.
- Clamshell: See earlier discussions.
- Lateral walk: See earlier discussions.

Day Three

The exercises should be performed as supersets, consisting of three sets with 12 to 15 repetitions each. Make sure the tenth repetition becomes challenging. The workout should take about 40 minutes.

- Standing wide row: See earlier discussions.
- Overhead press: See earlier discussions.
- Chest press: See earlier discussions.
- Band pull-apart: See earlier discussions.
- Biceps curl: See earlier discussions.
- Triceps kickback: Stand on a longish resistance band and bend forward from the waist. Hold the ends of the band in your hands and pull backward while in the bent position, reaching back as far as possible. For variety, you can try it with one arm at a time (BIQ Band Training, 2020).
- Lateral raise: See earlier discussions.
- High plank row: See earlier discussions.

Day Four

The exercises should be performed as supersets, consisting of three sets with 12 to 15 repetitions each. Make sure the tenth repetition becomes challenging. The workout should take about 40 minutes.

- Lying abduction: See earlier discussions.

- Hip thrust: See earlier discussions.
- Banded squat: See earlier discussions.
- Band-assisted pistol squats: See earlier discussions.
- Pull-through: See earlier discussions.
- Low-high chop: See earlier discussions.

Beginner Five or Six Day Workout

Are you ready to start your journey to fitness?

Keep the general background and guiding of the previous chapters in mind and listen to your body. While exercises should be challenging, they should not cause pain. Remember to warm-up properly and stretch and cool down afterward.

Prioritize the full range of motion in all exercises. Do it slower but all the way instead of trying to rush through the routine. Remember, this is dedicated time to yourself.

Adapt your goal to your current reality. Things that might have mattered to you twenty years ago are not so important anymore. Give yourself realistic reasons to show up for your home workout, and motivation will never be a problem, derailing your vision of a healthier and happier you.

Invest some time in learning meditation or tai chi, if you are so inclined. These mind exercises can be a great aid in visualizing the road ahead as well as the end result.

New experiences take time before you can get into your comfort zone, where they are easy. Give yourself that time and be kind to yourself; you're worth it.

Day One

This routine focuses on the lower body. The exercises should be performed as supersets, consisting of three sets with 12 to 15 repetitions each. Make sure the tenth repetition becomes challenging. The workout should take about 15 to 20 minutes with minimal breaks.

- Single-leg high extension: Anchor your band at waist height and feel it pull taut. Lift one knee as high as possible while pulling away from the anchor. For variety, you can lift the foot on the ground onto your toes at the same time (The Prehab Guys, n.d.).
- Pull-through: See earlier discussions.
- Glute bridge: See earlier discussions.
- Lying abduction: See earlier discussions.

Day Two

This routine is for the upper body. The exercises should be performed as supersets, consisting of three sets with 12 to 15 repetitions each. Make sure the tenth repetition becomes challenging. The workout should take about 15 to 20 minutes with minimal breaks.

- Bent-over row: See earlier discussions.
- Chest press: See earlier discussions.
- Overhead press: See earlier discussions.
- Side plank reach: See earlier discussions.

Day Three

This routine is for the lower body again. The exercises should be performed as supersets, consisting of three sets with 12 to 15 repetitions each. Make sure the seventh repetition becomes challenging. The workout should take about 15 to 20 minutes with minimal breaks.

- Single-leg deadlift: See earlier discussions.
- Split squat: See earlier discussions.
- Hip thrust: See earlier discussions.
- Bicycle crunch: See earlier discussions.

Day Four

An upper body routine today. The exercises should be performed as supersets, consisting of three sets with 12 to 15 repetitions each. Make sure the seventh repetition becomes challenging. The workout should take about 15 to 20 minutes with minimal breaks.

- Kneeling pull-down: See earlier discussions.
- Push-up: See earlier discussions.
- Arnold press: See earlier discussions.
- Side plank row: See earlier discussions.

Day Five

Today it is the turn of the full body. The exercises should be performed as a circuit, starting with the first exercise and ending with the last one, before going back to number one. The time for the workout should be about 20 minutes.

- Bent-over rear delt fly: See earlier discussions.
- Banded squat: See earlier discussions.
- Mountain climber: See earlier discussions.
- Overhead press: See earlier discussions.
- Hip raise: See earlier discussions.

Day Six

The whole body will again be exercised today. The exercises should be performed as supersets, consisting of three sets with 12 to 15 repetitions each. Make sure the seventh repetition becomes challenging. The workout should take about 15 to 20 minutes with minimal breaks.

- Chest press: See earlier discussions.
- Split squat: See earlier discussions.
- Face pull: See earlier discussions.
- High-low chop: See earlier discussions.

Advanced Five or Six Day Workout

Congratulations on getting this far, if you mastered the beginner routine first. You have progressed well on your way to a healthy, happy, and physically easier future.

For more advanced readers who start here, this program should provide enough of a challenge to get you moving. Use it as an example to put your own program together as it suits you.

Day One

These exercises are for the lower body. The exercises should be performed as supersets, consisting of three sets with 10 to 12 repetitions each. Make sure the tenth repetition becomes challenging. The workout should take about 40 to 50 minutes, with minimal breaks.

- Single-leg hip extension: See earlier discussions.

- Pull-through: See earlier discussions.
- Skater squats: See earlier discussions.
- Quadruped kickback: See earlier discussions.
- Glute bridge: See earlier discussions.
- Hip thrust: See earlier discussions.
- Banded squat: See earlier discussions.
- Torso rotation: See earlier discussions.

Day Two

Today we exercise the upper body. The exercises should be performed as supersets, consisting of three sets with 12 to 15 repetitions each. Make sure the tenth repetition becomes challenging. The workout should take about 40 to 50 minutes, with minimal breaks.

- Bent-over row: See earlier discussions.
- Chest press: See earlier discussions.
- Overhead press: See earlier discussions.
- Straight-arm pulldown: For variety on the arm pulldown exercise discussed earlier, you can keep your arms straight instead of bending them at the elbows. You could insert something like a light wooden rod in the loops of the band and place your hands at the ends of the rod instead of in the middle. That will keep your elbows wider and engage even more muscles (Rubberbanditz, 2019).

- Triceps press-down: To change the degree of difficulty from the exercise as discussed earlier, you could do this one arm at a time while keeping your core muscles tight and your back and ribcage straight (Showman, 2017).
- High curl: See earlier discussions.
- Mountain climber: See earlier discussions.
- Side plank reach: See earlier discussions.

Day Three

It is the lower body's turn again. The exercises should be performed as supersets, consisting of three sets with 12 to 15 repetitions each. Make sure the seventh repetition becomes challenging. The workout should take about 40 to 50 minutes, with minimal breaks.

- Single-leg deadlift: See earlier discussions.
- Split squat: See earlier discussions.
- Single-leg bench squat: See earlier discussions.
- Clamshell: See earlier discussions.
- Lateral walk: See earlier discussions.
- Hip thrust: See earlier discussions.
- Psoas march: See earlier discussions.
- Bicycle crunch: See earlier discussions.

Day Four

Time for the upper body to get a chance again. The exercises should be performed as supersets, consisting of three sets with 10 to 12 repetitions each. Make sure the seventh repetition becomes challenging. The workout should take about 40 to 50 minutes, with minimal breaks.

- Kneeling pull-down: See earlier discussions.
- Push-up: See earlier discussions.
- Arnold press: See earlier discussions.
- Band-assisted pull-up: See earlier discussions.
- Low biceps curl: Instead of standing in front of the band when pulling it towards you, you can lie down on the floor and pull the band from a low anchor. Keep your knees bent and your back and hips flat on the floor (Rubberbanditz, 2019).
- Overhead extension: See earlier discussions.
- Pec Fly: Also known as the chest fly exercise. See earlier discussions.
- Side Plank row: See earlier discussions.

Day Five

Today it is the turn of the full body. The exercises should be performed as a circuit, starting with the first exercise and ending with the last one, before going back to number one. The time for the workout should be about 36 minutes.

- Bent-over rear delt fly: See earlier discussions.
- Push-up: See earlier discussions.
- Banded squat: See earlier discussions.
- Glute bridge: See earlier discussions.
- Mountain climber: See earlier discussions.
- Overhead press: See earlier discussions.
- Biceps curl: See earlier discussions.
- Skater squats: See earlier discussions.
- Hip raise: See earlier discussions.

Day Six

The whole body will again be exercised today. The exercises should be performed as supersets, consisting of three sets with 12 to 15 repetitions each. Make sure the seventh repetition becomes challenging. The workout should take about 40 to 50 minutes with minimal breaks.

- Chest press: See earlier discussions.
- Split squat: See earlier discussions.
- Pallof press: Anchor your band firmly at shoulder height. Hold the end of the band in both hands against your chest. You can either stand or kneel, although the kneeling version is slightly more difficult. Step away from the anchor far enough that you can feel the band pulling you back. Straighten your arms towards the anchor and engage your core muscles to

stay upright with a straight back. Resist the band's attempts to get your torso to twist. Hold the position for as long as possible before relaxing (Coachmag, n.d.).
- Band-assisted pistol squats: See earlier discussions.
- Hip hinge: See earlier discussions.
- Single-leg bench squat: See earlier discussions.
- Face pull: See earlier discussions.
- High-low chop: See earlier discussions.

Your new habit and routines are started. Keep the momentum going, do not stop now. Your body and mind will thank you every day for the decision you took when you picked this book up, to invest time and effort in your health.

It is all about vitality and living your senior years with vigor. It is being able to experience the fullest range of functional movement possible given your specific situation.

Conclusion

Are you as excited as I am for you to start on the beautiful and rewarding road to a healthier, fitter, and happier version of yourself than you've ever been?

We started this journey of discovery looking at the what and the why of resistance bands. I told you a little bit about myself and my amazing experiences with exercise, as well as my passion for helping others to discover the same satisfaction and live their dream lives.

We looked at the benefits of exercise in general and uncovered its power and potential to prevent and heal certain illnesses and medical conditions. You learned all the reasons why resistance band training is an excellent way to harness the healing and rejuvenating properties of regular exercise.

I also introduced you to your new exercise companion, your set of resistance bands. Together we looked at the different types of bands available, the options they offer, and accessories that make them even more versatile. We briefly looked at some resistance exercises specific to golfers because there are so many seniors enjoying the sport. Golf is only one example of how bands can improve any game and prevent injuries.

You now know exactly what to do and what not to do for the best results. You have practiced some of the movements with me and experienced for yourself how much better you feel. You have seen for yourself how different exercises go together and complement each other for a whole body benefit. You have also acquired the know-how to compile your own workout routines to suit your circumstances and preferences perfectly.

A Final Piece of Advice

You have all the right knowledge and tools in your hands now, but it remains up to you to apply them to your life. You will not reap the success you desire if you do not make a commitment to yourself or a training partner to show up for regular workouts.

Your life is in your hands, and the choice is yours. Take the right decision and make today the first day of the new *You*!

It has been great fun to help you down this road of discovery. Thank you for allowing me to share my passion and some of my knowledge and experience. My biggest reward will be knowing that it transformed your life. Kindly leave a positive review of this book to let me know how it is working for you and so others can experience the improvements of having their own "fitness bible" on demand.

Do not go yet; One last thing to do...

If you enjoyed this book or found it useful I'd be very grateful if you'd post a short review on Amazon.com. Your support really does make a difference and I read all the reviews personally so I can get your feedback and make this book even better.

Thanks again for your support!

References

8fit Team. (n.d.). *8 Benefits of Resistance Bands and Two Workouts.* 8fit. https://8fit.com/fitness/resistance-band-benefits-and-workouts/

Alexander. (2011, August 12). *Don't Hold Your Breath - Suffocation will Affect your Workouts Negatively.* Fitzness.Com. http://www.fitzness.com/blog/dont-hold-your-breath-suffocation-will-affect-your-workouts-negatively/

Alternative Exercises Row. (n.d.). Your Body Programme. https://www.yourbodyprogramme.com/alternative-exercises-row

Alzheimer's Society UK. (n.d.). *Physical exercise and dementia.* Alzheimer's Society. https://www.alzheimers.org.uk/about-dementia/risk-factors-and-prevention/physical-exercise#:~:text=Combining%20the%20results%20of%2011

Amazon. (n.d.). *Grebest Heavy Duty Resistance Band, Pull UP Assist Bands Workout Resistance Bands for Body Stretching Powerlifting Mobility Single Band or Set.* Amazon. https://www.amazon.com/Grebest-Resistance-Powerlifting-Stretching-Weightlifting/dp/B079DNQTVT/ref=asc_df_B079DNQTVT/?tag=hyprod-20&linkCode=df0&hvadid=309821907754&hvpos=&hvnetw=g&hvrand=7597129508290966102&hvpone=&hvptwo=&hvqmt=&hvdev=c&hvdvcmdl=&hvlocint=&hvlocphy=9033326&hvtargid=pla-599317122411&psc=1

Amazon. (2020). *Amazon.com: RENRANRING Resistance Bands Set, Exercise Bands with Stackable Workout Bands, Door Anchor Attachment, Handles, Legs Ankle Straps, Carry Bag, Gym Equipment for Home (Set of 13) (Black): Sports & Outdoors.* Amazon. https://www.amazon.com/RENRANRING-Resistance-Stackable-Attachment-Equipment/dp/B08134VTJ6

Amazon Valeofit Store. (2020). *Valeo: Recovery*. Amazon. https://www.amazon.com/stores/page/692DC80A-844C-4D4E-B825-E950AE4275C8?ingress=2&visitId=c00a56a1-4f3d-4d1c-ada3-16ac48ea1907&ref_=ast_bln

Amazon.com: SUPERPUMP BFR BANDS | Simple + Effective Quick-Release Straps for Blood Flow Restriction Training and Kaatsu Style Workouts | Arms: Sports & Outdoors. (2020). Amazon. https://www.amazon.com/Superpump-Kaatsu-inspired-Training-Restriction-Maximum/dp/B01N45Z84Y

Andersen, C. (2014, July 10). *47 Crazy-Fun Plank Variations*. Greatist. https://greatist.com/move/plank-variations-for-core-strength#intermediate

Arana, J. (2019, March 29). *3 Ways to Perform Assisted Pull Ups - wikiHow Fitness*. Www.Wikihow.Fitness. https://www.wikihow.fitness/Perform-Assisted-Pull-Ups

Arnold Press - How To Do It. (n.d.). Move More Eat Better! http://www.exercise-guide-to-lose-weight.com/arnold-press.html

Atemi Sports. (2019, August 12). *15 Mini Resistance Band Ab Exercises for a Rock-Solid Core*. Atemi Sports. https://www.atemi-sports.com/mini-resistance-band-ab-exercises/

Barbara M. (2019, August 7). *Featured Exercise: Banded Pull-Throughs*. Barbell Strength. http://barbell-strength.com/banded-pullthrough/

Barber, E. (2018, December 11). *Get Fit with a Resistance Band*. Archery 360. https://www.archery360.com/2018/12/11/get-fit-with-a-resistance-band/#:~:text=Start%20by%20folding%20the%20band

Bentley, A. (2016, December 3). *Tip: Use Bands for Lateral Raises*. T NATION. https://www.t-nation.com/training/tip-use-bands-for-lateral-raises

BfR Professional. (2018). *Blood Flow Restriction Training- A complete guide*. BfR Professional. https://bfrpro.com/pages/blood-flow-restriction-training

BIQ Band Training. (2020, May 3). *Hip Thrust With Resistance Band*. BiqBandTraning.Com. https://biqbandtraining.com/hip-thrust-with-resistance-band/?v=7516fd43adaa

Biswas, C. (2018, April 25). *18 Best Resistance Band Exercises - Full Body Workouts*. STYLECRAZE. https://www.stylecraze.com/articles/resistance-band-exercises/#resistance-band-exercises-for-the-abscore

Bowden, J. (2015, October 9). *6 exercises using resistance bands for more distance.* Golf WRX. http://www.golfwrx.com/329714/6-exercises-using-resistance-bands-for-more-distance/

Brathwaite, P. (2018, February 9). *How to Perfect the Banded Curl.* Muscle & Fitness. https://www.muscleandfitness.com/workouts/arm-exercises/how-perfect-banded-curl-massive-biceps/

Cadman, B. (2020, January 24). *10 exercises to strengthen the lower back.* Www.Medicalnewstoday.Com. https://www.medicalnewstoday.com/articles/323204#lower-back-rotational-stretches

Callaway, M. (2018, December 7). *6 Psoas March Variations You Likely Haven't Tried Before |.* Meghan Callaway. http://www.meghancallawayfitness.com/my-blog/6-psoas-march-variations-you-likely-havent-tried-before/

Carpenter, H. (2020, May 21). *Use This Simple Progression to Work into a Pistol Squat.* Outside Online. https://www.outsideonline.com/2412982/how-do-pistol-squat

Chowdhury, M. H. (2019, September 22). *Best Resistance Bands For Seniors, And People Of Any Age For Bodybuilding.* Fitness of Body | Health and Fitness Tips, Healthy Food Habits Etc.

https://www.fitnessofbody.com/2019/09/best-resistance-bands-for-seniors-any-age.html

Coachmag. (n.d.). *How To Do The Pallof Press.* Coach. https://www.coachmag.co.uk/core-exercises/7392/how-to-do-the-pallof-press#:~:text=Engage%20your%20core%20and%20press

Collins, R. (2012, March 29). *Exercise, Depression, and the Brain.* Healthline. https://www.healthline.com/health/depression/exercise#:~:text=They%20help%20relieve%20pain%20and

Cordeau, B. (n.d.). *Lat Pulldown Loop Band.* Skimble. https://www.skimble.com/exercises/41947-lat-pulldown-loop-band-how-to-do-exercise

Creveling, M. (2020, June 18). *Can You Build Muscle Without Lifting Weights?* Shape. https://www.shape.com/fitness/workouts/bodyweight-training/build-muscle-bodyweight-exercises

Crowley, G. (2016, April 5). *Pilates – the importance of controlled movement.* Health Through Harmony. https://www.healththroughharmony.ie/pilates-the-importance-of-controlled-movement/

Cruz, N. (2019, June 7). *10 Ways to Get Stronger Without Lifting Weights.* LIVESTRONG.COM. https://www.livestrong.com/article/335541-

ten-ways-to-get-stronger-without-lifting-weights/

De Pietro, M. (2019, January 22). *Trapezius: Muscle pain, stretches, and home remedies.* Www.Medicalnewstoday.Com. https://www.medicalnewstoday.com/articles/324251

Dearden, K. (2017, December 13). *What are Therapeutic Resistance Bands?* Newcastle Sports Injury Clinic. https://www.newcastlesportsinjury.co.uk/what-are-therapeutic-resistance-bands/

Desertcart. (n.d.). *Shop brand renranring Online at Low Price in Botswana at botswana.desertcart.com.* Botswana. https://botswana.desertcart.com/brands/brand-renranring

Dick's Pro Tips. (2019, April 12). *Five Upper Body Resistance Band Exercises.* PRO TIPS by DICK'S Sporting Goods. https://protips.dickssportinggoods.com/sports-and-activities/exercise-and-fitness/five-upper-body-resistance-band-exercises

Dotfit. (n.d.). *Tennis Watcher. Dotfit.* https://www.dotfit.com/sites/63/images/articles/Exercise%20PDFs/Tennis%20Watcher.pdf

EDX USA. (n.d.). *Resistance.* EDX. https://edxusa.com/collections/resistance

EFM Healthclubs. (2018, October 19). *6 Benefits of Abdominal Workouts*. EFM Health Clubs. https://efm.net.au/benefits-of-abdominal-workouts/

Eisinger, A. (2019, November 8). *13 Super Effective Exercises That Work Your Arms, Back, and Shoulders*. SELF. https://www.self.com/gallery/arm-sculpting-slideshow

Fairview. (n.d.). *Neck Exercises: Head Lifts*. Fairview. https://www.fairview.org/sitecore/content/Fairview/Home/Patient-Education/Articles/English/n/e/c/k/_/Neck_Exercises_Head_Lifts_85975

Fanelli, L. (n.d.). *How to Use Resistance Bands for Strength Training*. Tomsofmaine. https://www.tomsofmaine.com/good-matters/healthy-feeling/how-to-use-resistance-bands-for-strength-training#:~:text=Simply%20stand%20on%20the%20band

Fetters, K. A. (2016, September 28). *Why Range of Motion Matters for Your Strength Training Goals*. Life by Daily Burn. https://dailyburn.com/life/fitness/strength-training-range-of-motion/

Fetters, K. A. (2019, December 27). *Why You Should Try the Windmill Exercise (and How to Do it)*. Openfit. https://www.openfit.com/windmill-exercise

Fit Carrots. (n.d.). *Core - Side Bends with Long Resistance Band*. FIT CARROTS | Premium Fitness Tools For Functional and Regeneration Training. https://www.fitcarrots.com/exercise/long-resistance-bands/core-side-bends-with-long-resistance-band/

Fitness Australia. (2018). *Resistance training – health benefits*. Better Health. https://www.betterhealth.vic.gov.au/health/healthyliving/resistance-training-health-benefits

Fort Healthcare. (2019, January 10). *Hand & Wrist Stretches for Computer/Smartphone Users*. Fort HealthCare. https://www.forthealthcare.com/hand-and-wrist-stretches-for-computer-and-smartphone-users/#:~:text=ceiling%20wrist%20stretch-

Freytag, C. (2014, July 12). *How To Use A Figure 8 Band*. Get Healthy U | Chris Freytag. https://gethealthyu.com/how-to-use-a-figure-8-band/

Garage Gym Reviews. (n.d.). *Best Tube Resistance Bands for 2020*. Garagegymreviews. https://www.garagegymreviews.com/best-tube-resistance-bands

Giacobbe, L. (2019, September 25). *How older adults can recover from exercise injuries.* Kendalathome. https://www.kendalathome.org/blog/bid/314169/how-older-adults-can-recover-from-exercise-injuries

Gomez, A. (2017, August 11). *This Tiny Tweak Will Take Your Mountain Climbers To The Next Level.* Women's Health. https://www.womenshealthmag.com/fitness/a19916561/fitgif-friday-mini-band-mountain-climber/

Gunsmith Fitness. (n.d.). *Hip Circles 101: Everything You Need to Know About This Unique Training Device.* Gunsmith Fitness. https://gunsmithfitness.com/blogs/news/hip-circles-101

Hagstrom, A. D., Marshall, P. W., Halaki, M., & Hackett, D. A. (2019). The Effect of Resistance Training in Women on Dynamic Strength and Muscular Hypertrophy: A Systematic Review with Meta-analysis. *Sports Medicine (Auckland, N.Z.), 50,* 10.1007/s40279-019-01247–x. https://doi.org/10.1007/s40279-019-01247-x

Harwood, R. (2018, March 22). *Resistance Band's with Handles VS without Handles.* Fitness Health. https://fitnesshealth.co/blogs/fitness/resistance-bands-with-handles-vs-without-handles

Health Benefits Of Physical Activity. (2019). MedicineNet. https://www.medicinenet.com/script/main/art.asp?articlekey=10074

Healthwise Incorporated. (2020, March 2). *Tennis Elbow | Senior Health Services*. Hhcseniorservices.Org. https://hhcseniorservices.org/health-wellness/health-resources/health-library/detail?id=hw225372&lang=en-us

HEB. (2020). *Protein Building Blocks*. H-E-B | No Store Does More. https://www.heb.com/static-page/article-template/Protein-Building-Blocks

Herman, D. (2017, October 16). *Benefits of Resistance Bands in Golf*. SuperFlex® Fitness. https://www.superflexfitness.com/benefits-of-resistance-bands-in-golf/

Hoffman, K. (2020, April 3). *9 Best Resistance Band Chest Exercises To Do At Home*. NOOB GAINS. https://noobgains.com/resistance-band-chest-exercises/

Iliades, C. (2019, May 13). *The Benefits of Strength and Weight Training | Everyday Health*. EverydayHealth.Com. https://www.everydayhealth.com/fitness/add-strength-training-to-your-workout.aspx

Jay, J. (2010, September 30). *Exercise Order - How To Arrange Exercises In Your Workout*. A Workout Routine.

https://www.aworkoutroutine.com/exercise-order/

Jewell, T. (2018, September 25). *Diaphragmatic Breathing and Its Benefits.* Healthline. https://www.healthline.com/health/diaphragmatic-breathing#benefits

Kamau, C. (2020, August 10). *Calorie Deficit But Not Losing Weight: What's The Culprit Behind It?* Weight Loss Blog - BetterMe. https://betterme.world/articles/calorie-deficit-but-not-losing-weight/#:~:text=Yes%2C%20it%20is.

Kassel, G. (2019, May 23). *How to Use Resistance Bands—Because You Know You Don't *Really* Know.* Shape. https://www.shape.com/fitness/tips/how-use-resistance-bands

Kelly, E. (2015, October 22). *What You Need to Know About Anaerobic Exercise.* Healthline; Healthline Media. https://www.healthline.com/health/fitness-exercise/anaerobic-exercise#benefits

Kelso, T. (n.d.). *The Top 5 Exercises to Strengthen Your Neck.* Breaking Muscle. https://breakingmuscle.com/fitness/the-top-5-exercises-to-strengthen-your-neck

Kendola, A. (2020, July 23). *8 lower back stretches for flexibility and pain relief.*

Www.Medicalnewstoday.Com. https://www.medicalnewstoday.com/articles/lower-back-stretches#knee-to-chest

Kilroy, D. S. (2014). *Exercise and Eating Healthy.* Healthline. https://www.healthline.com/health/fitness-exercise-eating-healthy

Knopf, K. (2010). *Healthy shoulder handbook : 100 exercises for treating and preventing frozen shoulder, rotator cuff and other common injuries.* Ulysses Press.

Kwon, Y. S., & Kravitz, L. (2019). *How Do Muscles Grow?* Unm.Edu. https://www.unm.edu/~lkravitz/Article%20folder/musclesgrowLK.html

Letsfit. (n.d.). *Fitness Accessories - Letsfit.* Www.Letsfit.Com. Retrieved October 20, 2020, from https://www.letsfit.com/product-list/110/Fitness_Accessories

Level, B., Sydney, 499 Kent St, & Email, N. S. W. 2000 A. +61 2 9267 5487. (2017, November 13). *15 Essential Foods You Need on a Fat Loss Diet - Ultimate Performance.* Ultimate Performance Sydney. https://up-australia.com/tips/15-essential-foods-need-transformation-diet/

Lori Michiel Fitness, Inc. (n.d.). *Choosing and using resistance bands in workouts for seniors.* Lori Michiel Fitness, Inc.

https://lorimichielfitness.com/resources/exercise-resistance-bands/

Lugo, J. (2017, August 15). *Lower Body Exercise: Skaters With A Mini-Band.* JLFITNESSMIAMI. https://juanlugofitness.com/lower-body-exercise-skaters-with-a-mini-band/

Lux Fitness. (n.d.). *Premium Booty Resistance Band Set.* Lux Retails. Retrieved October 20, 2020, from https://luxretails.com/products/hip-resistance-band-set

Marcin, A. (2018, February 12). *Tight Calves: Stretches, Treatment, Prevention, Causes, and More.* Healthline. https://www.healthline.com/health/tight-calves#causes

Mateo, A. (2017, October 9). *Legit Resistance Band Ab Workout.* Greatist. https://greatist.com/fitness/resistance-band-core-exercises-massy-arias#exercises

Matt. (n.d.). *How To Anchor Your Resistance Bands At Home: Easy and Cheap.* Home Gym Resource. https://homegymresource.com/how-to-anchor-your-resistance-bands-at-home-easy-and-cheap/

Maximum Training Solutions. (2016, July 20). *5 Variations of the Mini Band Sidestep.* Maximum Training Solutions -.

http://www.maximumtrainingsolutions.com/5-variations-of-the-mini-band-sidestep/

Mayo Clinic. (2016). *Osteoporosis - Symptoms and causes*. Mayo Clinic. https://www.mayoclinic.org/diseases-conditions/osteoporosis/symptoms-causes/syc-20351968

Mayo Clinic. (2018, December 18). *What you need to know about exercise and chronic disease*. Mayo Clinic. https://www.mayoclinic.org/healthy-lifestyle/fitness/in-depth/exercise-and-chronic-disease/art-20046049#:~:text=Regular%20exercise%20can%20help%20insulin

Men's Health. (2011, May 4). *You MUST Try This Ab-Blasting Exercise!* Men's Health. https://www.menshealth.com/fitness/a19529948/side-plank-and-row/

Merriam-Webster. (2011). *Definition of STRENGTH TRAINING*. Merriam-Webster.Com. https://www.merriam-webster.com/dictionary/strength%20training

Mirafit. (n.d.). *Top 8 Resistance Band Shoulder Exercises | Mirafit*. Mirafit.Co.Uk. https://mirafit.co.uk/blog/best-shoulder-exercises-using-resistance-bands/#:~:text=Tie%20the%20resistance%20band%20to

Mulrooney, M. (2011, July 8). *Figure 8 Resistance Band Exercises.* SportsRec. https://www.sportsrec.com/412995-figure-8-resistance-band-exercises.html

Murthi, A. M., & Ramirez, M. A. (2012). *Shoulder dislocation in older patients poses different challenges in diagnosis, treatment.* ScienceDaily. https://www.sciencedaily.com/releases/2012/10/121004134837.htm

National Posture Institute. (2014, March). *Why Postural Alignment is Important in Exercise Progression.* Www.Npionline.Org. https://www.npionline.org/articles/why-postural-alignment-is-important-in-exercise-progression

New Heights Physical Therapy. (n.d.). *The Three Phases of Healing | Portland OR & Vancouver WA.* New Heights Physical Therapy Plus in Portland OR Vancouver WA. https://www.newheightstherapy.com/phases-of-healing/

Newhouse, R. (2013, July 30). *The benefits of proper breathing during exercise.* MyNetDiary. https://www.mynetdiary.com/the-benefits-of-proper-breathing-during-exercise.html

NIAGARA LUTHERAN HEALTH FOUNDATION. (2016). *5 Benefits of Exercise for Seniors and Aging Adults | The GreenFields*

Continuing Care Community | Lancaster, NY. Thegreenfields.Org. https://thegreenfields.org/5-benefits-exercise-seniors-aging-adults/

No Foam Roller? No Problem! Try These Alternatives! | ISSA. (n.d.). Www.Issaonline.Com. https://www.issaonline.com/blog/index.cfm/2020/no-foam-roller-no-problem-try-these-alternatives

Nunez, K. (2018, August 16). *Need a Leg Press Alternative? 5 to Try*. Healthline. https://www.healthline.com/health/leg-press-alternative#resistance-bands

Patricie K. (n.d.). *Lying Band Back Fly*. Skimble. https://www.skimble.com/exercises/37666-lying-band-back-fly-how-to-do-exercise

Pedemonte, S. (2020, October 1). *How to Perform a Torso Twist*. Your House Fitness. https://www.yourhousefitness.com/blog/how-to-perform-the-torso-twist

Perfect Peach Athletics. (n.d.). *Perfect Peach Athletics - The #1 Fitness Brand for Women*. Perfect Peach Athletics. https://perfectpeachathletics.com/

Physioworks. (n.d.). *Exercise equipment – Physio Works*. https://physioworks.com.au/product-category/exercise-equipment/

Picincu, A. (2020, March 27). *Lawn Mowers and Back Exercise.* LIVESTRONG.COM. https://www.livestrong.com/article/336466-lawn-mowers-back-exercise/

Pridgett, T. (2019, June 15). *Burn Fat With This Cardio-Strengthening Bodyweight Exercise You Can Do Anywhere.* POPSUGAR Fitness. https://www.popsugar.com/fitness/How-Do-Resistance-Band-Sprints-46255833

Quinn, E. (2008, November 13). *How to Perform the Sit and Reach Flexibility Test.* Verywell Fit; Verywellfit. https://www.verywellfit.com/sit-and-reach-flexibility-test-3120279

Quinn, E. (2020, April 28). *What Exercises Help With ACL Rehabilitation?* Verywell Health. https://www.verywellhealth.com/acl-surgery-rehab-exercises-3120748

Rehabbing Sports Injuries with Resistance Bands. (2018, December 15). Prohealthcareproducts.Com. https://www.prohealthcareproducts.com/blog/rehabbing-sports-injuries-with-resistance-bands/

Resistance Band Lat Pulldown. (n.d.). Exercise. https://www.exercise.com/exercises/resistance-band-lat-pulldown

Resistance Band Lateral Raise. (n.d.). Exercise. https://www.exercise.com/exercises/resistance-band-lateral-raise

Rubberbanditz. (2019, February 6). *Chest Exercises with Resistance Bands*. Www.Rubberbanditz.Com. https://www.rubberbanditz.com/blog/chest-exercises-with-resistance-bands/

Rusin, J. (2017, June 14). *5 Ways To Make Face Pulls Even Better*. T NATION. https://www.t-nation.com/training/5-ways-to-make-face-pulls-even-better

Salyer, J. (2016, April 14). *Bridge Exercise: 5 Fun and Challenging Variations*. Healthline. https://www.healthline.com/health/fitness-exercise/glute-bridge-variations

Schrift, D. (2014). *How to Start With Exercises For The Elderly? Read on...* Eldergym®. https://eldergym.com/exercises-for-the-elderly/

Set for Set. (2017). *7 Rotator Cuff Resistance Band Exercises for Shoulder Rehab & Strength*. SET FOR SET. https://www.setforset.com/blogs/news/7-rotator-cuff-resistance-bands-exercises-for-rehab-prehab-and-strengthening

Set for Set. (2019, May 18). *What Size Resistance Bands Should I Get? Your Guide to Buying Bands*. SET FOR SET.

https://www.setforset.com/blogs/news/what-size-resistance-bands-should-i-buy

Sheppard, L. M. (2014). *How latex is made - material, production process, making, history, used, processing, components, composition.* Madehow.Com. http://www.madehow.com/Volume-3/Latex.html

Showman, N. (2017, September 14). *4 Resistance Band Exercises to Build Tricep Strength.* Muscle & Strength. https://www.muscleandstrength.com/articles/4-resistance-band-tricep-exercises

Simple Fitness Solutions. (n.d.). *Guidelines for exercise bands and exercise balls.* Simplefitnesssolutions. https://www.simplefitnesssolutions.com/resources/Guidelines.htm

Skimble. (n.d.). *Dumbbell Fly on Ball.* Skimble. https://www.skimble.com/exercises/2239-dumbbell-fly-on-ball-how-to-do-exercise

Snape, J. (2015, July 15). *Ectomorph, Endomorph And Mesomorph: How To Train For Your Body Type.* Coach; Coach. https://www.coachmag.co.uk/lifestyle/4511/ectomorph-endomorph-or-mesomorph-what-is-your-body-type

SoCal Health. (n.d.). *SoCal Health Group.* SoCal Health. https://socalhealthgroup.com

Soto, P. (2018, February 8). *The Single Leg Deadlift with a Resistance Band version*. Sports and Martial Arts in the United States and the Modern World. https://sportsandmartialarts.com/single-leg-deadlift-resistance-band-challenge/

Spark People. (n.d.). *Lying Abduction with Band Exercise Demonstration*. SparkPeople. https://www.sparkpeople.com/resource/exercises.asp?exercise=1

Starwood Sports. (n.d.). *Resistance Loop Band Exercise Guide*. Starwood Sports. https://uk.starwoodsports.com/pages/resistance-loop-band-exercise-guide

Sworkit Wellness. (n.d.). *Resistance Band Overhead Press*. Sworkit | At Home Workout and Fitness Plans. https://sworkit.com/exercise/resistance-band-overhead-press-2#:~:text=Stand%20on%20your%20resistance%20band

Taraniuk, L. (2019, July 22). *The importance of breathing during workouts*. Totalbalancehf. https://www.totalbalancehf.com/single-post/2019/07/01/The-importance-of-breathing-during-workouts#:~:text=When%20you%20exercise%20and%20your

The Definitive Guide to Resistance Bands and Workout Bands. (n.d.). WODFitters.

https://www.wodfitters.com/pages/the-definitive-guide-to-resistance-bands-and-workout-bands

The Movement Fix. (2018, September 3). *Standing Banded Row*. Movement Fix. https://themovementfix.com/standing-banded-row/

The Prehab Guys. (n.d.). *Double Leg Hip Hinge With Resistance Band*. **[P]Rehab**. https://theprehabguys.com/vimeo-video/double-leg-hip-hinge-with-resistance-band/

The right way to warm up and cool down. (2019, July 9). Mayo Clinic. https://www.mayoclinic.org/healthy-lifestyle/fitness/in-depth/exercise/art-20045517#:~:text=A%20warmup%20gradually%20revs%20up

Theraband. (n.d.). *About Us - TheraBand*. Www.Theraband.Com. Retrieved October 20, 2020, from https://www.theraband.com/about-us

Timco Rubber. (n.d.). *Rubber Extrusion Process, Extruded Rubber Process*. Timcorubber. https://www.timcorubber.com/rubber-resources/rubber-extrusion-process/

Tinsley, G. (2017, October 1). *How to Improve Body Composition, Based on Science*. Healthline. https://www.healthline.com/nutrition/improve-body-composition#TOC_TITLE_HDR_4

Train With Me Fitness Inc. (n.d.). *Train Online Signup*. Trainonline. https://www.trainonline.com/reverse-band-woodchops-exercise

Tribe Fitness USA. (n.d.). *Resistance Bands*. Tribe Fitness. https://www.tribefitnessusa.com/collections/resistance-bands

University of Birmingham. (2018). *A lifetime of regular exercise slows down aging, study finds*. ScienceDaily. https://www.sciencedaily.com/releases/2018/03/180308143123.htm

University Orthopedics. (n.d.). *University Orthopedics - Foot and Ankle Exercises*. University Orthopedics. https://universityorthopedics.com/educational_resources/foot_exercises.html#:~:text=Ankle%20Stretch

Upham, B. (2018, April 6). *The Possible Way Strength Training Reduces Insulin Resistance | Everyday Health*. EverydayHealth.Com. https://www.everydayhealth.com/type-2-diabetes/treatment/mechanism-strength-training-can-help-reduce-insulin-resistance/

Victoria, A. (2016, October 25). *No clue how to foam roll? Watch this!* TODAY.Com. https://www.today.com/health/foam-rolling-5-minute-routine-stretch-your-body-t104297

Waehner, P. (2019, November 21). *Turn Your Exercise Ball Into a Strength Training Machine.* Verywell Fit. https://www.verywellfit.com/total-body-workout-with-bands-on-the-ball-1230909#:~:text=Chest%20Press

Watkins, W. (2014, December 19). *Fitness Fix: Strengthening Your Pelvic-Floor Muscles.* Experience Life. https://experiencelife.com/article/fitness-fix-strengthening-your-pelvic-floor-muscles/

WebMD. (n.d.). *What Is Trochanteric Bursitis?* WebMD. Retrieved October 13, 2020, from https://www.webmd.com/pain-management/trochanteric-bursitis#1

WebMD. (2007). *Runner's Knee: What You Need to Know.* WebMD; WebMD. https://www.webmd.com/pain-management/knee-pain/runners-knee#1

Weight Loss Resources UK. (n.d.). *Upper Body Muscles.* Weightloss Resources. https://www.weightlossresources.co.uk/exercise/muscles/upper_body.htm

Weingart, H. M., & Kravitz, L. (2020). *Resistance Training and Bone Mass.* Unm.Edu.

https://www.unm.edu/~lkravitz/Article%20folder/bonemass.html#:~:text=There%20is%20increasing%20emphasis%20on

What is Thermoplastic Rubber? (TPR). (2017, September 5). KMA SA Marketing. https://www.kmasa.co.za/thermoplastic-rubber-tpr/

Whatafit. (n.d.). *Whatafit - Shenzhen Yongming Wangluokeji Youxiangongsi.* Whatafit. http://www.whatafit.net/

Wheeler, T. (2019, December 18). *Slideshow: Benefits of Strength Training.* WebMD. https://www.webmd.com/fitness-exercise/ss/slideshow-benefits-strength

Williams, L. (2020, March 6). *Use the Quadruped Hip Extension to Build Better Glutes.* Verywell Fit. https://www.verywellfit.com/how-to-do-a-quadruped-hip-extension-4685857

Williamson, L. (2019, December 12). *Consistency Is The Most Important When Training For Muscle Growth.* Www.Womenshealth.Com.Au. https://www.womenshealth.com.au/consistency-most-important-factor-for-building-strength-muscle-growth-resistance-training

Winderl, A. M. (2017, June 27). *13 of the Best Exercises for Your Side Abs.* SELF.

https://www.self.com/gallery/obliques-exercises

YMCA of the North. (n.d.). *Long-term benefits of regular exercise*. YMCA of the North. https://www.ymcanorth.org/blog/2017/04/04/5991/long_term_benefits_of_regular_exercise

Young, L. (2020, February 27). *4 Key Body Parts You Should Exercise Now*. Best Health Magazine Canada. https://www.besthealthmag.ca/best-you/fitness/main-body-parts-to-work-out/

Ziftex. (n.d.). *Products*. ZIFTEX. https://ziftex.com/collections/all

Images

Ashram, S. (n.d.). Seniors on yoga mats. In *Unsplash*. https://unsplash.com/photos/QgCl-pNkfPc

Canburn, L. (n.d.). Woman on fitness ball. In *Unsplash*. https://unsplash.com/photos/f4RBYsY2hxA

Henry, M. (n.d.-a). Resistance band leg stretch. In *Burst*. https://burst.shopify.com/photos/resistance-band-leg-stretch?q=resistance+bands+workout

Henry, M. (n.d.-b). Tensor squat band. In *Burst*. https://burst.shopify.com/photos/tensor-band-squats?q=loop+resistance+bands

Mars, B. (n.d.). Women with resistance bands. In *Unsplash*. https://unsplash.com/photos/oLStrTTMz2s

Pflug, S. (n.d.). Women with flexible bands, ready to do a chest press. In *Burst*. https://burst.shopify.com/photos/woman-strong-band-exercise?q=resistance+bands+workout

Pieters, G. (n.d.). Exercising with resistance bands. In *Unsplash*. https://unsplash.com/photos/3RnkZpDqsEI

Shopify Partners. (n.d.). Tubular resistance band. In *Burst*. https://burst.shopify.com/photos/fitness-product-squat-band?q=tubular+resistance+bands

Sikkema, K. (n.d.). Resistance tubing. In *Unsplash*. https://unsplash.com/photos/rWBBDErPXcY

Van, D. (n.d.). Resistance bands. In *Unsplash*. https://unsplash.com/photos/Mzu7qcmP5tk

© Copyright 2020 by

FRANCIS PAPUN

All rights reserved

www.ingramcontent.com/pod-product-compliance
Ingram Content Group UK Ltd.
Pitfield, Milton Keynes, MK11 3LW, UK
UKHW020720270225
4780UKWH00021B/524

9 781777 314088